GW00713207

Coleman, Dr V

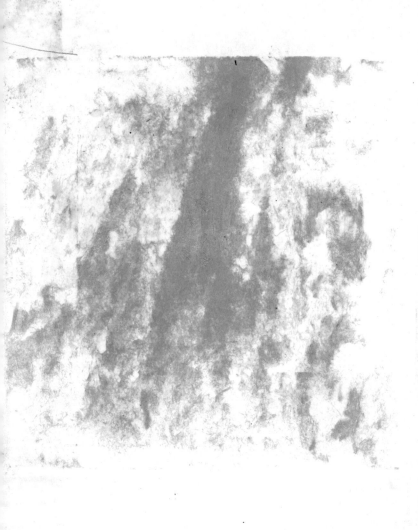

Eczema and Dermatitis

Other books by the same author

On Medicine

The Medicine Men
Paper Doctors
Everything You Want To Know About Ageing
Stress Control
The Home Pharmacy
Aspirin or Ambulance
Face Values
Stress and Your Stomach
Guilt
The Good Medicine Guide
A Guide To Child Health
BodyPower
An A-Z of Women's Problems
Bodysense
Taking Care of Your Skin

On Cricket

Thomas Winsden's Cricketing Almanack
Diary of a Cricket Lover

As Edward Vernon

Practice Makes Perfect
Practise What You Preach
Getting into Practice
Aphrodisiacs – An Owner's Manual
The Complete Guide to Life

Other books in this series

High Blood Pressure
Diabetes
Arthritis

Dr Vernon Coleman's
healthbooks
for all the family

ECZEMA
and
DERMATITIS

by

DR VERNON COLEMAN

SEVERN HOUSE PUBLISHERS

This first world edition published 1985 by
SEVERN HOUSE PUBLISHERS LTD, of
4 Brook Street, London W1Y 1AA

British Library Cataloguing in Publication Data

Coleman, Vernon
   Eczema and dermatitis: Dr. Vernon Coleman's
   medical handbooks for all the family.
   1. Eczema
   I. Title
   616.5'21   RL251

   ISBN 0-7278-2077-X Cased
   ISBN 0-7278-2057-5 Pbk

To Tony and Gertrude,
dear friends

Printed and bound in Great Britain by
Butler & Tanner Ltd, Frome and London

Contents

Note

This book is not intended as a substitute for the medical advice of physicians. The reader should consult a physician in all matters relating to health and particularly in respect of any symptoms that may require diagnosis or medical attention. While the advice and information here are believed to be true and accurate at the time of going to press neither the author nor the publisher can accept any legal responsibility or liability for any errors or omissions that may have been made. The inclusion of the names of companies, associations and products in this book does not imply any endorsement by the author, and the omission of names of companies, associations and products does not imply any criticism or lack of faith.

The various forms of eczema and dermatitis make up more than half of all the skin disorders seen in general practice.

Fact-file on eczema

Eczema or dermatitis

There is a good deal of confusion about the difference between the two words 'eczema' and 'dermatitis'. Rather than create two definitions and add to the confusion I have chosen to regard the two words as identical and to use the single word 'eczema' throughout.

What are the symptoms?

'Eczema' is not a single disease: it is a skin problem, caused by a number of different factors, but usually showing itself by a well-defined set of symptoms.

These are:
    dryness
    redness
    itchiness
    swelling
    blistering
    weeping

Some or all of these symptoms may be present and the significance of different symptoms can vary a good deal. The skin often looks raw, sore and uncomfortable. The fluid that has leaked from the blistered skin may dry to form a crust. Because the area itches a lot it tends to get scratched. And that means that infection is quite a common complication.

Is it infectious?

No. There are no forms of eczema which are infectious. Confusion may be caused because eczema does often run in families.

So several people in the same household may have a similar looking rash.

Will eczema last for life?

Not necessarily. When babies and children develop eczema there is a very good chance indeed that their skin condition will improve over the years.

Do all eczema sufferers also suffer from asthma?

No. There is a link between asthma, hay fever and eczema – they are often all allergy problems. But although babies and children who suffer from eczema do seem to have an increased chance of developing asthma in later life the link is by no means inevitable.

What causes eczema?
Genetics

Some types of eczema do seem to be inherited. Atopic eczema, for example, is likely to run in a family. When one parent has atopic eczema then the risk of a child having an allergy problem of some kind (eczema or asthma) is approximately fifty per cent. If both parents have atopic eczema then the chances of a child being affected are higher still.

The genetic factor is only one influence. An individual can develop eczema when there is no family history of the disorder and, equally, you can have perfectly healthy skin even though there is a strong family history of eczema.

When there is a family history of eczema it is worthwhile taking care to reduce the risk of other influences causing it. It is, for example, sensible to take care to protect the skin against the sun, wind, rain and cold.

Personality

During recent years, researchers all around the world have been trying to find out whether or not there is any fundamental difference between the sorts of individuals who develop peptic ulcers, the types who get high blood pressure and the sorts who end up with eczema.

It is, after all, relatively rare for one individual to suffer from more than one major disease problem. So it is reasonable to assume that some physical or mental characteristic must decide which particular problem will affect an individual.

The evidence which has been accumulated so far suggests that the most important factor is personality.

Psychologists and psychiatrists and trained observers of all kinds now claim that it is possible to predict just what sort of person ends up with asthma, arthritis or depression. This information is invaluable for two reasons.

First, because we know what sort of individuals get asthma (for example) we can pick out those individuals, and help them reduce their risks of developing that particular problem. It isn't possible to change anyone's personality, of course, but it is often possible to adapt or alter one's attitudes, habits and behavioural patterns. And, of course, it is also possible to reduce other risk factors. So, for example, with someone whose personality marks them as an asthma risk, avoiding cigarettes is a priority.

Second, once an individual has been diagnosed as suffering from a particular ailment (such as eczema) it is often possible to help that individual get better by teaching him how to adapt his approach to life. If your personality, attitude and approach to life have caused a specific problem then by altering them you can often solve or lessen that problem.

The following list of traits is not intended to provide a pen picture of all eczema patients, of course. It is unlikely that any one patient will fit perfectly into the pattern that has been recorded (and indeed, it is possible for an individual who has none of these personality traits to develop eczema for there are, of course, factors other than personality involved).

However, if you are a sufferer look through the list and see whether or not you recognise yourself or your own behavioural patterns. Later on (see pages 58-62) I will include some advice on just how to adapt your attitudes to help your skin condition.

● Many eczema sufferers tend to be extremely sensitive

individuals who repress their emotions. So, for example, when you are upset or sad you may refuse to cry and refuse to let other people see just how upset you really are. This sort of attitude is particularly prevalent among males who will almost certainly have been taught as boys to suppress their emotions.

• Eczema sufferers often tend to be dependent. As children they will probably have been given a lot of attention when ill but treated strictly when fit. It is easy for parents to fall into this trap. It is natural to be generous and kind to a child with inflamed, sore skin. And it is equally natural to be keen to balance this with a little strictness when the child is feeling better. The trouble is that the eczematous child who is treated in this way tends to grow up to associate love and affection with poor health and dependence. Parents should try to be consistent in their dealings with their child.

• You are probably sensitive to stress. For years many people have been bewildered by the fact that some individuals seem to cope extremely well with enormous amounts of stress and others crack up when the stress levels are still modest. The truth is that we all respond differently to stress and we all have different stress thresholds. It is not the amount of stress we are subjected to which causes the problems so much as our ability to cope with that stress. If you have a fairly low stress threshold then you are likely to suffer even if your job and home life are relatively peaceful. Just missing a bus or finding that a button has come off a shirt will be enough to cause you worry and anxiety. If you have a high stress threshold you will be able to cope perfectly well with circumstances which might put someone else in hospital. Do not worry if you do have a low stress threshold, however. Even if you do over-react to stress there is still much that you can do to protect yourself. (See pages 62-68.)

• You probably carry more guilt than is your fair share. Like people who suffer from asthma, eczema patients tend to be particularly unselfish and loyal. They worry a lot about what other people think.

• You are almost certainly a worrier. You probably worry about just about anything and everything that comes your way. You worry about whether or not you are going to have enough

13

money (even if you have enough for your needs); you worry about whether you are doing a good job; about whether the people close to you are happy. And you worry about your skin problem.

Do remember that not all eczema sufferers will exhibit all these personality traits. But look through the list and see if any of them apply to you. Then you can find out how to adapt your personality so that you can cope effectively without making your skin condition worse. And do remember too that I am not suggesting that any of the traits here are bad ones. Some of these are traits which make you a good, reliable, honest individual. These are not traits which need to be eradicated. But when problems such as eczema develop they may well need controlling a little.

Stress

One of the most important reasons for the high incidence of eczema these days is the fearful increase in the amount of stress with which we all have to cope.

That may sound a strange claim for two reasons.

First, how can such a nebulous, ill-defined force such as stress cause a visible change in the state of the skin?

And second why should we, in our modern homes, suffer from stress at all? After all, most of us have plenty of food to eat, we have somewhere warm and dry to sleep every night and we do not have to worry too much about being attacked or eaten by wild animals. Compared to our ancestors we would, on the surface, appear to have an easy time of it. You would not really think that we were much more likely to suffer from stress-induced diseases than our ancestors, would you?

Let us look at those two points in turn.

First, how can stress affect the state of the skin? To answer this question you have only to remember that the skin is an important vehicle for emotional expression. When we are frightened we turn white; when we are embarrassed we go red; when we are anxious our sweat glands work overtime and our skin becomes sweaty and slippery. It is, it seems, always the skin which knows first when there is any confrontation between the body and its environment.

Second, we suffer so much from stress simply because our bodies were not designed for the sort of stress we have to endure these days. We were designed for an instant world.

If you turn a corner and come face to face with a man-eating tiger then your body will react remarkably effectively to that instant threat.

Your heart will beat faster in order to ensure that as much blood as possible reaches your muscles (this ensures that plenty of oxygen reaches the tissues which may have to work extra hard to get you out of the scrape); acid will pour into your stomach (this ensures that any food there will be converted into usable energy and reach your blood stream as speedily as possible); and your muscles will tense (to ensure that you are well prepared for fighting the tiger, running away from it or climbing up the nearest tree).

There will also be a change in the amount of blood flowing to your skin. The vital organs need to be well supplied and it is safer to keep the amount of blood flowing through the skin to an absolute minimum in case of injury. It could be that the reduced blood flow to the skin explains the dryness that is so common among eczema sufferers, and which is thought to be a precursor to the ailment.

In the sort of physical world our ancestors lived in a few thousand years ago that sort of response would have helped to keep them alive. If you could run, fight and climb then you had a good chance of surviving. Those traits were handed down from father to son simply because the individuals who were not good at running, jumping, climbing and fighting (in other words the individuals whose muscles did not tense and whose hearts did not beat faster) were all eaten by wild, marauding animals.

Unfortunately, in our modern world those natural, automatic responses are not always appropriate. Indeed, they are sometimes a hindrance rather than a help.

The trouble is that we have changed our world far quicker than our bodies have been able to evolve. Revolutionary changes in agriculture, navigation, medicine, science, military tactics, industry and so on have changed the world a great deal. These days there are not many man-eating tigers around. And most of our threats and problems cannot be solved by physical action.

The simple truth is that we have changed our world too much. Our bodies have just not been able to cope. Today we respond to danger in exactly the same way that our ancestors responded thousands of years ago. But today the dangers and threats are different.

These days we do not have to worry about being eaten: we have to worry about paying our bills, keeping our jobs, coping with inflation, fighting off court summonses, policemen and traffic wardens, and dealing with the million-and-one administrators and bureaucrats who impinge on our lives.

Our bodies respond to these modern threats in exactly the same way that they would have responded to the man-eating tiger: the heart beats faster, the blood pressure goes up, the skin goes white, the muscles become tense, and so on.

Unfortunately, these responses, although perfectly natural, are quite inappropriate.

If you have bills to pay, a job to find or a parking ticket to pay, those natural, physiological responses will not help you at all. Increased muscle tension and a higher blood pressure will help you run or fight. A reduction in the amount of blood flowing into your skin will protect you against a possible blood loss. But those responses will not help you deal with piles of paperwork or officious administrators.

Worse still, because our modern problems tend to go on and on for long periods, the natural stress responses remain switched on and our muscles stay tense and our hearts continue to beat faster for months or even years. Similarly our skin remains deprived of essential blood supplies. What was intended as a protective response, and a temporary one at that, has become a damaging one.

Understand all this and it becomes easy to see why stress is one of the main causes of eczema. It is also easy to see why it is important for anyone who suffers from it to learn how to cope with stress.

Is stress affecting your skin condition?

Some people are much more susceptible to stress than others. While one individual will be able to cope perfectly well with an apparently endless series of major crises, another will be sent into a state of panic at the thought of missing a train or the sight of a button coming off a shirt. Our stress thresholds vary enormously and so it is helpful to know just how vulnerable you are to stress. If you have a high stress threshold you will be able to cope with tremendous pressures. If, on the other hand, you have a low stress threshold then you will need to minimise your exposure to stress if you want to keep your eczema under control.

To benefit from the quiz that follows you must answer all the questions – and answer them accurately.

1 Do you get physical symptoms such as headaches, indigestion, vomiting or diarrhoea before important meetings or appointments?
   a always
   b never
   c sometimes

2 When you are anxious or excited, does your:
   a pulse race and your heart pound?
   b your pulse increase a small amount?
   c your pulse stay much the same as usual?

3 If you are concentrating hard on what you are doing and someone suddenly comes up behind you, do you:
   a jump a mile?
   b respond involuntarily but quickly get control of yourself?
   c remain calm and unperturbed?

4 When you are frightened or anxious or upset, does your face:
   a stay much the same as usual?
   b go a little pale?
   c go quite white?

5 When you are upset or nervous, do you:
   a get butterflies in your stomach and sweat a good deal?
   b get just one of those symptoms?
   c get neither of them?

6 What is your reaction time like?
   a below average
   b average
   c above average, very fast

7 Do you ever have difficulty in breathing when you are excited?
   a often
   b occasionally
   c never

8 When you become angry or furious, does your face:
   a stay the same as usual?
   b redden a little?
   c go bright red?

9 If you are waiting for an important phone call which does not come, do you:
   a become a nervous wreck?
   b get a bit edgy?
   c remain quite calm?

10 If, when you are lying in bed at night, you are suddenly woken by an unexpected noise, do you:
   a wake up quickly and completely?
   b take ages to wake up and realise what has happened?
   c wake up quite quickly but take a few seconds to realise exactly what has happened?

Now add up your score.

1	a3 b1 c2		**6**	a1 b2 c3
2	a3 b2 c1		**7**	a3 b2 c1
3	a3 b2 c1		**8**	a1 b2 c3
4	a1 b2 c3		**9**	a3 b2 c1
5	a3 b2 c1		**10**	a3 b1 c2

If you scored between 20 and 30 then you are the sort of individual who would survive well in a world where physical dangers posed a threat. You would stand a good chance of surviving in the jungle, for example, where your fast reactions would help you look after yourself. On the other hand, you are not, I am afraid, well suited for our modern world. And your skin problem is likely to have been caused or made worse by the way that you respond to stress. You will probably be able to improve the condition of your skin by learning to avoid excessive stress, and by learning to increase your capacity to cope with stressful situations.

If you scored between 13 and 19 then you are very much in the middle range, between the two extremes. You would probably still benefit from learning how to control your responses to stress.

If you scored 12 or less you would not probably last long in the jungle or in any sort of environment where physical threats are common. But you are fairly well adapted to life in the modern world. It is unlikely that your eczema has been caused by your responses to stress.

Diet and eczema

There has, in recent years, been much discussion about the link between food and eczema. A number of sufferers have claimed that they have been able to get rid of their skin symptoms simply by changing their diet and either cutting out one particular type of food or eating large quantities of another.

The foods most often described as causing eczema include: eggs, cheese, cows' milk, fish, chicken, wheat, sugar and food colourings and preservatives. Although I have no doubt that the patients who make these claims have evidence to show that their dietary rules work, there is no convincing clinical evidence to show that dietary changes can affect all cases of eczema. It is likely that only those patients whose eczema is of the allergic type will benefit. (See page 26.) And they will only benefit when they manage to find the specific food to which they are allergic.

The one link that has been established is that between babies, cows' milk and eczema. Breast feeding does seem to reduce the chances of eczema developing in a child.

If you feel that your eczema could be caused by something in your diet there are two possible ways to tackle the problem. First, if you suspect that you know the food that is causing the problem, simply cut it out of your diet. (Cows' milk and eggs seem to be the two most likely culprits.) Avoid it for at least five days, and then see if there is any improvement. You may need to stay off the food for longer than that to obtain a result. You may, incidentally, feel a little 'odd' while on your exclusion diet. It is possible to develop a food addiction alongside a food allergy – so there may be some strange withdrawal symptoms.

If, however, you have no idea of the nature of the food likely to be causing your eczema, or you have tried cutting out cows' milk and eggs and obtained no useful result, I suggest you ask your doctor to help you follow a proper exclusion diet.

I do not recommend following any strange or unusual diet. You are more likely to produce problems than to relieve symptoms. Speak to your doctor first. It is, of course, particularly important not to put children on any sort of exclusion diet without medical advice.

Kitchen hazards

The kitchen can affect eczema sufferers in two ways.

First, most people will probably agree that they often fail to dry their hands properly after doing kitchen chores. If you are busy doing the dishes and the telephone rings, you will probably make do with a perfunctory wipe on a rather soggy, threadbare kitchen towel. This can lead to a number of skin problems but in particular it can cause a loss of natural skin oils and moisture. That means the skin becomes extra dry and that, in turn, means an exaggerated risk of developing or exacerbating eczema. A good supply of fresh, soft towels kept near all the sinks in your house will help your skin tremendously. If you cannot acquire proper towels then get a supply of paper kitchen towelling.

Second, and equally hazardous, is the tendency to plunge bare hands into bowls full of hot water laced with detergent, bleach or some other powerful chemical. All chemicals are potentially harmful and many which we use in the kitchen can do a great deal of damage to the skin. (It is worth remembering, by the way, that hot water in itself is more damaging than cold water.)

Anyone who suffers from eczema or dry skin should take care to use cotton lined rubber gloves (and if surgeons can do heart transplants while wearing rubber gloves then I am sure that most people should be able to do the dishes in rubber gloves). Make sure that you buy gloves that are large enough to get on and off without too much trouble. You can buy ridged rubber gloves these days and they reduce the risk of your dropping valuable and much treasured items of crockery. Long handled kitchen mops are also extremely helpful. I sometimes think that doctors should be able to prescribe these two items for regular eczema sufferers.

Finally, of course, it is well worth remembering that if you have dry or sensitive skin or you suffer from eczema then you should definitely use a barrier cream to protect your hands when working in the kitchen. And you should keep a tub of moisturising cream near to the sink.

Air conditioning – a menace rather than a boon

Theoretically, modern air conditioning is designed to control the amount of moisture in the atmosphere, the temperature, the movement of fresh air supplies and the number of impurities in the air. That, in theory, is the idea and there is little doubt that if air conditioning systems all worked efficiently then we would all benefit.

Unfortunately, many air conditioning systems are so badly designed, or so badly run, that they are more of a menace than a help. The biggest problem with them is that they tend to dry the air too much and that increases the risk of catarrh and sinus problems developing and it tends to make normal skin dry and cracked. If the air around you is dry, water will evaporate from your skin.

You can help yourself in a number of ways. First, you can try and persuade someone to deal with the air conditioning system. Turning it off altogether may be the only answer. Commercial humidifiers will sometimes deal with the dryness or you can put a large bowl of water on the floor. Or you could even drape wet towels or clothes over radiators. As a last resort you can try opening the windows.

If you find yourself in these circumstances make sure that you use a good moisturising cream. Keep a pot of your favourite moisturiser with you at work and take a small pot with you wherever you go.

The weather

Whether it is wet or dry, sunny or cloudy, the weather can have an adverse effect on your skin.

When it is cold, for example, the blood supply to the surface of your skin will be restricted so that your body will lose a minimum amount of heat. This reduction in blood flow means that your skin will be deprived of essential moisture and essential nutrients. It will be more likely to become dry and cracked.

The wind has an adverse effect on your skin too. In just the same way as a good breeze will be welcomed by anyone trying to dry wet clothes on a washing line so a breeze should be regarded with some suspicion by anyone with dry skin. For the wind can take water from your skin in the same way that it takes water from wet clothes.

Then there is the rain. You only have to look around in our big cities to see the sort of damage done to our older buildings by the acid-rich rain that has been falling for the past few decades. Rain that can eat through stone can also do your skin a good deal of harm.

And finally, of course, there is the sun.

We all tend to be enthusiastic about sunbathing these days, and desperately keen to acquire fashionable tans. What we often forget is that when the skin turns brown it is trying to protect itself from the effects of the sun, since the ultra-violet light emitted by the sun can cause changes in the structure, chemistry and function of the skin's tissues. Sunshine is partly responsible for the ageing process that affects our skin and this is why the hands and the face are usually wrinkled, dry and papery before other parts of our bodies. Most of us expose our hands and faces to more sun than, say, our buttocks, upper arms and thighs.

When white or pink skin is exposed to the sun a number of things happen. To begin with skin cells are injured and they release a histamine type of substance which produces reddening and itching of the skin. After a period of time, which may vary from hours to days, cells deep inside the skin start to release a substance called melanin which slowly migrates towards the surface. Melanin is the pigment which gives the skin its tan and its purpose is to provide some protection against further damage. Dark skinned people already have a protective layer of melanin on the outer skin surface and they can sunbathe with relative impunity. (Although even if you have dark skin you should still use a moisturising cream to stop your skin getting too dry.)

Those are not the only effects which the sun has on human skin. There is also a severe drying effect, and the skin becomes tougher and thicker too. The thickening blocks the skin's pores and the drying up leads to a shedding of powdery white particles made up of dead cells. Blood vessels dilate as a result of the heat and fluid may leak out into the tissues giving the skin a tight, swollen look and feel to it. Blisters and peeling are common sequels. All these harmful changes can lead to the development of eczema or worsen an existing condition.

The damage that the sun can do to the skin depends on a number of factors which are worth mentioning.

The skin type is obviously important since, as I have already pointed out, darker skinned individuals are already protected to a certain extent (the extent depends on the colour of their skin). Fair haired or red haired people with light blue eyes and pale, freckled skin are the most susceptible and most likely to develop skin problems.

The intensity of the sun, and the amount of time spent in the sun, are also vital factors. Latitude, altitude, season, time of day and the surrounding environment all affect its strength. The sun is more dangerous when it is high in the sky, when the sunbather is near to the equator or when the air is thin and relatively unpolluted as it is on mountain slopes.

Snow, water, sand and white buildings all reflect the sun's

rays and make it stronger. And, of course, you should also remember that you do not have to sunbathe to be exposed to the sun. Sportsmen and sportswomen usually age quicker than people who spend all their time in nightclubs away from the sunshine. An outdoor existence may be a healthier existence in many ways but as far as your skin is concerned an indoor life is better.

The single most important thing that you can do to protect yourself against all these different weather hazards is to apply a moisturising cream.

Sunbeds

In order to supplement their holiday sunshine many people are now using sunbeds during the winter months. Thousands of sunbeds have been bought for private use and there are countless private clinics where you can rent a sunbed for half an hour or so.

Buying time on a sunbed is a good way to buy skin trouble.

Lying on a sunbed is just as dangerous as spending time in the sun. There is a risk of being burnt and there is a real risk of your skin becoming too dry. (There will always be exceptions and I am quite prepared to believe that there will be readers who can claim that their eczema has been helped by time on a sunbed. I accept this possibility but would still argue that, on balance, using a sunbed is not wise for people with skin problems.)

Incidentally, it is probably worth knowing that only about one in three people get a good suntan from lying on a sunbed. The other two thirds either end up with a moderate tan or with no tan at all. It seems that there are differences between the type of suntan obtained from ordinary sunshine and the type obtained from a sunbed. People who normally tan well in the sun do not necessarily tan well on a sunbed and a sunbed tan will not always prevent burning when you are exposed to the sun.

As you will have probably guessed I am not too fond of sunbeds. My dislike of them is based partly on clinical experience with patients and partly on scientific papers which condemn sunbeds.

24

Occupational hazards

Occupational eczema is the commonest type of job-related disease in the Western world. More than half the people who suffer from an illness caused by their work suffer from a skin problem.

Obviously it is too huge a task to produce a comprehensive list of all the chemicals and irritants likely to cause dermatitis or eczema. Nor is it possible to produce a list of all the types of work which might lead to eczema. It would probably be easier to produce a list of jobs and chemicals which do not carry a risk of eczema.

Whether you work in a hairdressing salon or a factory, an office or a bank, a shop or a hospital then I am afraid you are at risk. Eczema can be caused or made worse by detergents, antiseptics, polishes, foods, bleaches, cleansers, solvents, oils, soaps, metals, rubber, creams and even by water.

If you suspect that your eczema is caused or made worse by the work that you do then answer the following questions:

• Does anyone else at work suffer from a skin problem? It does not have to be an identical problem to yours. But if there are two of you working in similar conditions with similar substances and you both have a skin problem then there is a very good chance that a job-related irritant is responsible.

• Does your eczema improve when you are away from work on holiday, or during the weekend? If it does then that suggests that it is a result of something that you are in contact with at work.

• Does your skin problem come and go as you change your job at work? So, for example, if you always work with one particular type of product during the first week of every month and you always get a skin problem at that time then it is likely the two are related.

• Does your eczema only affect certain parts of your body that are exposed to irritants? The hands are most likely to come into contact with irritant substances. But it is sometimes possible for there to be a less instantly apparent link. So, for example, if you are a mechanic working with oil you may protect your hands with a base cream and with rubber gloves. But if you then wipe your oil laden hands down the front of your work trousers the oil may seep through the trousers and produce a rash on your legs. It is perfectly possible for eczematous rashes on the feet, back, chest, arms and even genitalia to be caused like this.

● Has your union or trade organisation any record of job related skin disease? If there is a genuine risk of developing eczema because of what you do then your union will almost certainly know about it. And they will also know about any steps you can take to protect yourself. Remember that your employer has a responsibility to protect you against job hazards.

Quick guide to the main types of eczema

Eczema can be caused in all sorts of ways. In practice it is more or less impossible to differentiate neatly between the different types of eczema (the guide that follows is intended to offer a simple explanation to the various terms used, rather than a definitive dictionary of eczematous conditions). The whole picture is frequently confused by the fact that it is perfectly possible for a single case of eczema to be a mixture of several different types of eczema. So, for example, a child who has an inherited susceptibility to eczema may suffer as a result of an irritant which has been in contact with his skin. Mixed forms of eczema are extremely common and make it difficult for anyone to produce confident diagnoses.

Allergic eczema

Eczematous skin rashes can be caused by eating types of food or by swallowing drugs to which an allergy response has been acquired. Almost any foods can cause allergic eczema but the most likely ones are eggs and dairy produce. Penicillin and sulphonamide, two popularly prescribed anti-infective drugs, are perhaps the commonest pharmacological causes of allergic eczema.

Allergic contact eczema

If someone becomes allergic to a particular substance then he will develop symptoms of eczema on contact with that substance. When an attack of eczema is caused by an allergy reaction to a specific substance the skin symptoms are identical to those which occur in irritant eczema (see page 28). The commonest causes of allergic contact eczema are nickel, rubber, sticking plaster, chemicals and household plants.

Allergic contact eczema can be investigated by patch testing. (See page 78.)

Atopic eczema

This is the commonest type of eczema among young children. It usually develops between the ages of three months and two years. It tends to start on the face and nappy area, later spreading to the neck, hands, wrists and the fronts of the arms and legs. Atopic eczema usually gets better when the child reaches the age of four or five.

There is firm evidence to show that this type of eczema is less common in children who have been breast fed than in children who have been fed on cows' milk. Many experts now believe that atopic eczema is seven times as common in children who have been bottle fed as it is in children who have been fed with breast milk.

Discoid eczema

Also known as nummular eczema, discoid eczema consists of round, coin-shaped patches of eczema. There is usually some crusting around the edge of each patch and scaling in the centre. There is some confusion as to why eczema should develop in this way although it seems likely that there is some infective component.

Drug-induced eczema

Drugs taken by mouth can produce eczema (see Allergic eczema) but it is also important to remember that some creams and ointments (particularly steroid creams and ointments) prescribed for the topical treatment of eczema can exacerbate the condition.

Endogenous eczema

Endogenous or constitutional eczema is caused by some problem within the body rather than by some outside influence. For instance, an inherited allergy.

Exogenous eczema

Eczema produced by a reaction between the skin and some outside agent. Contact eczema is an exogenous eczema.

Infected eczema

Because eczematous skin is exposed and raw it can easily get infected. Many different types of infection – including bacteria, fungi and parasites such as scabies – may be involved. Before infected eczema can be treated the infection must be identified.

Inherited eczema

A phrase sometimes used as an alternative to atopic eczema.

Irritant eczema

Irritant eczema develops through a simple irritation of the skin. In babies and small children, for example, the commonest cause is the dribbling of saliva across the chin. Nappy rash, caused when urine soaked nappies stay in contact with the skin for too long, is another example. The commonest irritants are soap, water and detergents and just about anyone can develop irritant eczema. People who spend a lot of time with their hands in water (at the kitchen sink, for example) are particularly prone to develop it.

Light-induced eczema

Also known as photosensitive eczema this skin problem usually affects the face and the backs of the hands and other areas often exposed to the sun. The chances of developing light-induced eczema seem to increase after taking certain drugs or using chemicals which sensitise the skin. (See page 73.)

Seborrhoeic eczema

Seborrhoeic eczema affects mainly the scalp and usually looks like bad dandruff. The redness and scaling can spread away from the scalp and involve the hairline, the eyebrows, the nose, the ears and even further down the body.

Unclassified eczema

It is often impossible to decide just why a particular case of eczema has developed. It is then sometimes described as un-classified.

Varicose eczema

Varicose eczema usually affects the skin on the legs and is associated with varicose veins. The poor supply of blood to the skin and the pooling of stale blood in the veins produces a typical eczematous rash.

Doctors and drugs:

medical treatments for eczema

The role of the general practitioner

Although he may not be able to make a firm diagnosis, telling you the precise cause of your eczema, and although he may not be able to eradicate your symptoms entirely, your doctor has an important part to play in the treatment of your skin problem.

He can help you with advice, he can prescribe drugs that are only available on prescription and he can, when necessary, make an appointment for you to see a skin specialist (or dermatologist).

There is a great deal that you yourself can do to help keep your eczema under control. But you must work in partnership with your family doctor.

Getting the best out of your doctor

Far too many patients come out of a doctor's surgery and *then* remember that they have forgotten to tell him something that was vitally important − or to ask something they really needed to know.

There are many explanations for this, of course. First, most people worry about their health. That is perfectly natural. So, when they need to see a doctor they tend to be nervous and anxious. It is hardly surprising that they forget what they wanted to say. And, second, the advice that doctors give can be complicated and involve such things as when and how to use creams, when to return to the surgery, what side effects to watch out for, and so on and so on.

I think that when you are going to see your doctor you should plan your visit carefully, and before going sit down for a few minutes and try to think of everything that you want to tell your doctor – and everything you want to ask him. Then note it all down on a piece of paper.

You must, obviously, tell him about any symptoms you have. Tell him not just about the ones that seem important to you but of everything else you may have noticed too. Something that seems irrelevant to you may provide a vital clue.

On your first visit to the surgery tell him about any close relatives who also have skin problems, and be prepared to answer questions about your job, your hobbies, your eating habits and your personal medical history. If you have a past history of any disease you must tell him about it. Your doctor may have forgotten or the information may be hidden in your files. Your doctor will probably want to know about any family history of asthma, hay fever or other allergy problems.

It is also wise to tell him about any pills, tablets or creams that you are already using; whether they are products that have been prescribed or products that have been bought over a chemist's counter. You must even tell him if you have been borrowing someone else's cream or ointment. That may well have an influence on what he decides to offer you.

Remember, too, to jot down any specific questions that you want to ask. You may want to know whether you can carry on swimming. Or whether you should carry on doing the washing up even when wearing rubber gloves.

Write down all the questions you want answered. Obviously, if you go in to see your doctor clutching a huge three hundred-page account of your medical history and you have hundreds of questions to ask then he is going to become a little impatient. But he will not mind at all if you go in with a few notes jotted down. Indeed, he will almost certainly appreciate the fact that you are trying to make his job easier.

And write down the advice he gives you. If he tells you about your pills make a note of what he tells you. Make a note about the dosage, about any possible side effects, about when to stop taking the pills, about whether or not you need to avoid any particular foods or alcohol while on the drugs. Remember too to make a note about advice concerning the way to use creams or ointments.

Make a careful note about when you have got to go back to the surgery, about whether or not you need to see anyone at the hospital and, if you do need to see a specialist, the name of the doctor he is referring you to.

Doctors write down everything you tell them. And there is absolutely no reason at all why you should not write down everything the doctor tells you.

The role of the hospital specialist

You should always ask for an appointment with a dermatologist (skin specialist) if your eczema seems to be uncontrolled or you are unhappy with the treatment you are receiving from your general practitioner.

Most of the time skin specialists prescribe the same sort of creams, ointments and pills as general practitioners. But they do have access to more sophisticated forms of investigation and they will undoubtedly know of new forms of therapy being tried out and have access to hospital beds. If your symptoms are particularly bad a dermatologist may want you to stay in hospital for a day or two so that he can try a concentrated form of treatment.

Drug treatments for eczema

Scores of different products are prescribed for eczema sufferers. Most of the products available do, however, fall into a small number of categories.

MOISTURISERS
Now that the hazards associated with the over-use of steroid creams have been recognised, more and more doctors are prescribing simple moisturisers. There is a lot of evidence to show that such simple creams and ointments can often help relieve the symptoms associated with eczema and, indeed, improve the condition itself.

Simple moisturisers usually contain substances such as liquid paraffin, lanolin oil, soya oil, calamine, white soft paraffin, wool fat, and zinc oxide.

BARRIER CREAMS (also known as protective creams)

Barrier creams are insoluble and inactive and simply cover the skin in order to protect it from potential irritants. They usually contain dimethicone or a similar silicone oil. Barrier creams may produce allergy reactions.

ANTI-INFECTIVE PREPARATIONS

There is a wide variety of anti-infective creams available; some containing antibiotics and designed to deal with bacterial infections; some containing anti-fungal agents and designed to help deal with fungal infections.

Penicillin and sulphonamide are not normally used on the skin because there is a high risk of an allergy reaction developing. For the treatment of bacterial infections it is usual to select a cream which contains one of these antibiotic drugs: neomycin, bacitracin, framycetin and polymixin B.

For the treatment of fungal infections creams containing nystatin or griseofulvin are usually selected.

ANTI-PRURITIC SKIN PREPARATIONS (anti-itching)

In the past a number of different creams and ointments were used to help relieve itching. Unfortunately, it is now known that local anaesthetics and anti-histamine creams are both likely to produce allergy reactions. They are not, therefore, widely used. Calamine lotion, an old fashioned remedy, is one preparation that is safe and has survived. Otherwise, most doctors trying to deal with itching will either prescribe a moisturiser or an anti-histamine tablet.

CORTICOSTEROID PREPARATIONS (steroid creams and ointments)

When the human body needs to control internal inflammation it produces its own supplies of corticosteroid hormones.

Because the corticosteroids are good at controlling inflammation, doctors use synthetic versions of these hormones to help them deal with all sorts of inflammatory disorders within the body. So, for example, steroids given by mouth or injection are used to deal with such disorders as arthritis and asthma.

Unfortunately, it is now known that although the corticosteroids are natural drugs, they do have a number of dangerous side effects when used in large, unnatural quantities.

Sadly, the same thing is true of the corticosteroid skin preparations. They are powerful, extremely effective but potentially dangerous.

A number of points must be remembered when corticosteroid skin preparations are being used:

1   Corticosteroids do not cure any skin problems; they merely suppress the symptoms. This means that if the underlying skin problem does not clear up by itself, or is not dealt with in some other way, then when the steroid preparation is stopped the original symptom will eventually return. Corticosteroid preparations merely provide temporary relief.

2   When corticosteroids are used the resistance to infection is lowered. This means that anyone who uses a steroid cream for a long period of time on an area of inflamed skin will stand an increased chance of developing a skin infection.

3   Corticosteroids can sometimes delay the rate at which ulcerated or raw skin heals.

4   If corticosteroid creams are used for long periods of time they can flatten and thin the skin, producing scarring and marking. There will be some stretching of the skin too and it will sometimes look papery and old.

5   Your skin can become 'hooked' on steroid creams. If you use a steroid cream regularly and you want to stop using the cream then you will need to wean yourself off the product slowly under your doctor's supervision. If you are using a powerful steroid cream then you will need gradually to change to weaker and weaker versions.

6   If too much steroid cream is used for too long then the cream can be absorbed into the blood stream and can produce damaging side effects throughout the body.

7   In order to ensure that the cream remains potent and uninfected it is important to ensure that you always put back the top firmly. (This advice should, of course, be followed for all creams, ointments, and skin preparations.)

8 Eczema often improves during pregnancy, but if it does not it is important to be careful when using a steroid cream. Excessive use could increase the risk of your developing stretch marks and it might possibly damage your baby.

9 When applying a steroid cream use as little as possible. Smear the cream directly onto the eczematous area and do not rub it in. Make sure you know how many times a day you should be using the cream. You will probably be using your steroid cream only once a day.

10 Steroid creams are not intended for long term use. They are extremely useful and effective for the short term control of eczema.

11 If you have been given a steroid cream but your skin condition changes then visit your doctor so that he can check the suitability of the prescription. If, for example, your skin becomes infected then it may be necessary for him to prescribe a cream that contains both a steroid and an anti-infective of some kind.

12 You should be cautious about using steroid creams, but not afraid of them. They play an important part in the care and treatment of eczema.

There are scores of different corticosteroid preparations on the market, but only a limited number of basic steroid ingredients. Hydrocortisone is the safest and most widely used drug and is usually available in strengths ranging from 0.1% to 2.5%. Most hydrocortisone products fall within the range 0.25% to 1.0%.

Many steroid preparations do, however, contain a fluorine side chain – and are known as fluorinated corticosteroids. These tend to be more potent than hydrocortisone preparations. Fluorinated corticosteroids usually contain one of these constituents: betamethasone, fluocinolone and fluocortolone. There are, however, many other fluorinated corticosteroids available.

When using a corticosteroid preparation you should try not to use more than 50 grams a week; you should not continue for more than two weeks without consulting your doctor, and you should not obtain the drug without seeing your doctor (in other words you should not obtain the steroid on a 'repeat prescription' – a prescription obtained without consultation with your doctor).

ANTIHISTAMINE DRUGS

Antihistamines help to control allergy reactions and help eczema patients by controlling itching.

The main disadvantage with antihistamines is the drowsiness that usually accompanies their usage. For this reason you should take particular care if prescribed them. Do not drive or operate any machinery or go swimming or cycling until you are certain that you are not going to be affected. Because of this factor antihistamines are useful for controlling itching at night.

Although usually prescribed as tablets, antihistamines are also available in liquid form.

There are, of course, many other drugs used in the treatment of eczema. Antibiotics may need to be given by mouth if a patch of eczema becomes badly infected, disinfectants and antiseptics may sometimes be required and occasionally tar preparations will be used.

Getting the best out of prescribed drugs

Drugs, whether they are prescribed in tablet form or as creams or ointments to be applied to your skin, can be dangerous. But they can also be extraordinarily useful. To get the best out of drugs, while at the same time minimising the risks you run, you need to know how to use drugs safely and effectively. Read through the following notes.

● Always make sure that you find out as much as you can about the drugs that you have been given. If your doctor does not tell you when your drugs need to be taken then ask him for information – he may forget to put the advice on your prescription. The most important things you need to know are:

1 For how long the drug needs to be used. If you have been prescribed a special cream or ointment you should know whether you are to keep on using the product even after your skin has improved.

2   How much to use. If you have been prescribed a cream or ointment then you should try and get some idea of just how much you should use on each occasion. Should you use a generous dollop or a small smear? And should you try to rub it into your skin until it disappears or should you just leave it lying on the surface?

3   How many times a day a medicine should be used. If a tablet needs to be taken once a day then it does not usually matter what time of day it is taken as long as it is taken at the same time of day.

    If a drug has to be taken twice a day then it should be taken at intervals of twelve hours. A drug that needs to be taken three times a day should be taken at eight-hourly intervals (unless you are instructed otherwise) while a drug that needs taking four times a day should be taken at six-hourly intervals. Modern drugs are powerful and sophisticated; they need to be taken at exactly the right time if the right effects are to be obtained.

4   How the drugs should be taken in relation to meals. If you are taking tablets find out whether they should be taken before meals, during meals or after meals. Some drugs may cause stomach problems if taken on an empty stomach – they will obviously be safer if taken with food. Other drugs are not properly absorbed if taken with food.

● When you have been given instructions about how to use a drug make sure that you follow the instructions carefully.

● Remember that many drugs do not mix well with alcohol. It is always safer to assume that you should not drink while taking a drug until you have checked with your doctor.

● You must not take non-prescribed medicines while taking prescribed medicines. Nor must you use non-prescribed creams or ointments while using creams or ointments that have been given you by your doctor. The effects of different drugs can often be changed quite dangerously by mixing them.

● Occasionally, drugs do not mix with foods. If your doctor tells you not to eat a particular type of food then it is important that you follow his instructions.

● Keep all drugs in a locked cupboard where the temperature is stable. Although most of us keep our medicines in the bathroom that really is not the best place for them – the temperature and humidity levels there tend to vary too much. Your bedroom is probably best.

● Do not remove drugs from their proper containers except when you are taking them or when you are transferring them to a special 'day' box to carry around with you.

● Some drugs prescribed for eczema sufferers can cause drowsiness. If you have to drive a motor car or handle any machinery then it is particularly important that you ask your doctor if the drugs he has prescribed will have this side effect.

● Never ever take drugs or use creams or ointments that have been prescribed for someone else. Even if they seem to have the same symptoms as you, their medication may not suit you. Similarly, you should always resist the temptation to lend your drugs to someone else. And do remember that this is just as true of creams and ointments as it is of pills and potions.

● It is important that once you start receiving treatment you always try to see the same doctor. If several doctors are prescribing for you the chances are that your drug regime will become complicated, chaotic and confusing. Different doctors prefer different remedies for the treatment of eczema. It is also important to see the same doctor each time because only then will a proper assessment of your progress be able to be made.

● Be on the look out for side effects and do remember that if you seem to develop a second illness then the chances are high that it is caused by the treatment for the first.

Remember too that even creams and ointments can cause uncomfortable side effects and may themselves produce rashes and skin problems that look very much like eczema.

Reading your prescription

Unless your doctor dispenses his own drugs you will usually be given a prescription. You will be expected to take that prescription along to a local pharmacy where your drugs will be made up.

On that prescription will be written all the instructions that the chemist needs.

The name of the drug will be there, of course, together with instructions about when the drug is to be taken, whether it is to be taken with meals or before them, and so on.

Normally, those instructions should be written on the label of the bottle you are given. But, occasionally, some instructions are omitted. And that can lead to confusion.

To avoid that risk I have here included a list of the Latin abbreviations used by doctors when writing prescriptions, together with their meanings.

Now you can read your own prescription for your eczema medication.

Abbreviation	Latin	English
aa	*ana*	of each
ac	*ante cibum*	before meals
ad lib	*ad libitum*	freely
alt die	*alt diebus*	alternate days
alt noct	*alt noctibus*	alternate nights
aqua calida	*aqua calida*	hot water
bal	*balneum*	bath
bd	*bis in die*	twice a day
bid	*bis in die*	twice a day
c	*cum*	with
cat	*cataplasma*	a poultice
cc	*cum*	with
cm	*cras mane*	tomorrow morning
cn	*cras nocte*	tomorrow evening
dol urg	*dolore urgente*	when the pain is severe
eq	*equalis*	equal
ex aq	*ex aqua*	in water

Abbreviation	Latin	English
ext	*extractum*	extract
f	*fiat*	let it be made
flav	*flavus*	yellow
fol	*folium*	leaf
fs	*semi*	half
ft	*fiat*	let it be made
gutt	*guttae*	drops
haust	*haustus*	draught
hn	*hac nocte*	tonight
hor decub	*hora decubitus*	at bedtime
hs	*hora somni*	at bedtime
m	*misce*	mix
m et sign	*misce et signa*	mix and label
m ft mist	*misce fiat mistura*	mix and let a mixture be made
md	*more dicto*	as directed
midu	*more dicto utendus*	to be used as directed
mist	*mistura*	mixture
mit	*mitte*	send
om	*omni mane*	every morning
on	*omni nocte*	every evening
paa	*parti effecti applicandus*	to be applied to the affected part
p oc	*pro oculis*	for the eyes
prn	*pro re nata*	when needed
pulv	*pulvis*	powder

Abbreviation	Latin	English
qd	*quater in die*	four times a day
qh	*quatis horis*	four hourly
qid	*quater in die*	four times a day
qq	*quaque*	every
qqh	*quarta quaque hora*	every fourth hour
qs	*quantum sufficiat*	as much as is sufficient
r	*recipe*	take thou
rep	*repetatur*	let it be repeated
rep dos	*repetatur dosis*	let the dose be repeated
si dol urg	*si dolor urgeat*	if the pain is severe
sig	*signetur*	let it be labelled
sig	*signa*	label
sos	*si opus sit*	if necessary
ss	*semi*	half
stat	*statim*	immediately
syr	*syrupus*	syrup
td	*ter in die*	three times a day
tds	*ter die sumendum*	three times a day
tert qq hora	*tertia quaque hora*	every third hour
tid	*ter in die*	three times a day
ung	*unguentum*	ointment
ut dict	*ut dictum*	as directed

Essential glossary

Skin preparations are described in many different ways – confusing as it all may be it is important to know the difference between a cream and an ointment, a base and an application.

ANTISEPTIC An antiseptic is any agent that is designed to kill small organisms. For practical purposes the word 'antiseptic' is pretty much interchangeable with the words 'germicide' and 'disinfectant'. Many manufacturers put antiseptics into all sorts of different products – suggesting that by using them it is possible to cleanse the skin of bacteria. That is all nonsense I am afraid. You are not likely to be able to get rid of all the bacteria from your skin simply by using an antiseptic cream.

BARRIER CREAM A thick, protective cream which contains a high proportion of oil. Barrier creams are very useful if you suffer from dry or sensitive skin or if you work with chemical irritants of any kind.

BASE A base is a bland substance, usually a very plain and simple cream, that has no medicinal qualities of its own. Pharmacists use base creams when preparing medicated creams and ointments which are going to have to carry active substances. Base creams are also used to dilute preparations containing such active ingredients as hydrocortisone.

COLD CREAM A thick, cleansing cream which contains a very high proportion of oil and is therefore quite greasy to the touch.

CREAM A cream is merely a medical substance that has the consistency of the oily part of milk. Creams tend to spread much easier than ointments which, in comparison, tend to be sticky and messy.

EMOLLIENT An application which is rubbed onto the surface of the skin in order to help soothe and relax it as well as the tissues underneath.

EMULSION A mixture of two immiscible liquids, one being dispersed throughout the other in small droplets.

LINIMENT An oily preparation designed to be rubbed onto the skin.

LOTION A liquid preparation which may have modest medicinal qualities but is usually intended to soothe or protect the skin.

MOISTURISER A moisturiser protects your skin in the same way that a piece of waxed paper keeps sandwiches fresh. Although the word moisturiser suggests that something is put into the skin it actually works by preventing the loss of moisture that is already there. Most moisturising creams on the market contain a mixture of two substances: oil and water. The thickness and texture of the cream depends on just how much oil and how much water there is in the preparation. At one end of the scale there are the vanishing creams. These contain a relatively large amount of water and a small amount of oil and as their name suggests they more or less disappear entirely when rubbed onto the skin. Cold creams are at the other end of the scale.

NOURISHING CREAMS You are not likely to have a nourishing cream prescribed by your doctor. But you may see advertisements for them in magazines and newspapers. The manufacturers sometimes claim or suggest that by using their special product you will be able to 'feed' your skin. I am afraid this is nonsense. Anything fed into the skin is absorbed into the bloodstream.

OINTMENT Ointments are greasier, stickier and messier than creams but they are useful on dry, crusty skin. Ointments often contain one or more medicinal substances such as antiseptics, antibiotics or steroids.

PAINT In medicinal terms a paint is any medicament designed to be applied to the surface of the skin with a brush.

PASTE A paste is a semi-solid preparation which is even firmer and stickier and messier than an ointment.

POULTICE A soft, usually rather squashy mass which is served up warm and placed directly onto the skin as a counter irritant. It is a rather old fashioned (but nevertheless effective) way to soothe a sore or inflamed part of the body.

POWDER A host of tiny particles obtained by grinding a solid mass. Pharmacists use a mortar and pestle to make powders but factories do it on a rather larger scale.

SHAKE LOTION A rather convenient way to apply powder to the skin. The water in which the powder is suspended evaporates, cooling and soothing the skin as it goes, and leaving the powder behind. Because it consists of an insoluble powder suspended in water a shake lotion needs to be shaken before use. Shaking is much more effective than stirring by the way. Calamine lotion is a good example of a shake lotion.

VANISHING CREAM A cream which can be rubbed onto the skin without leaving a trace. A vanishing cream usually consists of a small amount of oil and a large amount of water.

Eczema control programme

Introduction

There is much that you can do yourself to help your eczema. You may not be able to cure your symptoms or even do away with the need to use steroid creams. But you will almost certainly be able to reduce your symptoms, improve the quality of your life and reduce your dependence on prescribed drugs.

Look after your skin

We all need to take care of our skin. But for eczema sufferers skin care is especially important.

If you read the beauty pages of popular magazines or you look at the advertisements prepared by companies selling skin products then you will probably become confused about just what you really need to do in order to protect your skin. Study what the so-called 'beauty experts' have to say and you will end up believing that you need to spend a fortune to provide yourself with any useful protection. I am pleased to say this is not true. Many of the 'beauty experts' talk absolute nonsense when it comes to discussing skin care. They repeat the slogans of the cosmetic companies because they simply do not know any better, and they happily regurgitate all sorts of pseudo-scientific nonsense in an attempt to convince you, the reader, that they know what they are talking about.

So let us start right at the beginning with the nature of skin itself.

It is here that the pseudo-science immediately gets out of hand. There are the writers talking about the importance of opening up the skin's pores, the journalists advocating the unique qualities of avocado oil and the beauticians highlighting the importance of respecting the skin's acid mantle. Listen to their claims and suggestions with cynicism and scepticism. People who talk or write in such terms almost certainly know less about skin care than you do.

Consider, for example, the question of skin type.

Most experts seem inclined to divide skin into four main types: normal, dry, oily and combination. There are, however, those who take themselves even more seriously who have added 'sensitive', 'slightly dry' and 'moderately oily' to this classical quartet.

To help you find out just what sort of skin you have got the beauty industry has developed all sorts of clever little tests. They suggest that you feed information into their special computers, they tell you to try sticking bits and pieces of tissue paper onto your skin and they tell you to peer at yourself closely in the mirror.

Then, they say, you will be able to find out which bits of your body have which types of skin. Once you have done that then they will be happy to sell you all the necessary ingredients to keep your skin healthy and strong.

It is all balderdash.

Your skin is not necessarily always dry or greasy any more than your nose is always clear or stuffy. You may have a tendency towards dry skin or you may have fairly greasy skin but I think it is silly and misleading to try and fit people into categories. We are all different and our skin conditions change all the time according to the way we feel, according to our health and according to the nature of our environment. If you are an eczema sufferer then you *probably* have a tendency to suffer from skin that is too dry. And you *probably* have skin that is exceptionally sensitive. But although those factors may influence some aspects of your lifestyle I do not think they really need influence your general skin care programme.

There are certain basic rules of skin care which apply to all types of skin.

Traditionally skin care falls into three basic categories: cleansing, toning and moisturising. I will deal with these three areas of skin care in turn.

Cleansing

First, cleansing. This is an essential part of your daily skin care. If you want to keep your skin healthy then you have got to cleanse it properly. The basic aim is to remove environmental dirt and unwanted cosmetic preparations. It is important that this is done without irritating the skin.

The number of products available for skin cleansing is vast. Different manufacturers recommend different types of soap, liquid soap, cleansing soaps, cleansing milks, cleansing liquids, detergents and so on. I have even seen bars of soap described as cleansing bars.

Ordinary soap is often dismissed as crude and dangerous by beauticians who want to sell you something more exotic and far more expensive. Take no notice. The purpose of any cleansing operation (that is the sort of technical term used by beauticians for a procedure most of us know as 'having a wash') is to remove dirt. And soap, when used with water, is particularly good at doing this.

Unless you know that a particular type of soap makes your skin worse, do not be afraid to go for the ordinary brands.

Just what sort of soap to buy is more difficult. There are probably hundreds of different types of soap available these days. There are, for example, the transparent soaps. These cost more than ordinary soaps because they are slightly more difficult to make. However, I have not been able to find any evidence to suggest that they are any better for your skin than non-transparent soaps. Nor do I think it worth your while buying triple or hard milled soaps, or super fatted soaps. Although these are sometimes said to be better for dry skins than ordinary soaps there is no real evidence to show that this suggestion is based on fact.

In addition to the basic, ordinary types of soap there are many soaps that contain extra ingredients. There are, for example, many types which contain perfumes and deodorants. I really cannot see any point in buying soaps which contain perfumes since when you are washing it is important that you wash off all traces of the soap afterwards. Adding extra perfumes merely increases the risk of your developing an allergy reaction.

There are, too, the soaps that contain 'medicated' ingredients. These are sometimes recommended for preventing skin infections. You can safely ignore these claims. Indeed, you should never buy any skin product described as 'medicated'. It is probably more expensive and more dangerous than a non-medicated equivalent product.

Since it is now known that the skin is normally slightly acid (whereas soaps are usually fairly alkaline) there are soaps said to be specially designed to maintain the skin's normal acid mantle. This is another attempt to part you from your money without offering you any real, long lasting benefit. You really cannot change the acid mantle of the skin merely by switching soaps.

The silliest types of soap are the ones that are said to moisturise your skin while they cleanse it. How can you possibly clean your skin properly while at the same time adding moisturiser? The companies who sell soaps which moisturise will probably be selling soaps which contain your make-up next. It would make about as much sense.

Nor, incidentally, is it worth your while spending extra money on liquid soaps. These tend to be more expensive than solid soaps and there is no reason why they should be safer or better for your skin.

In conclusion, you should use the cheapest, simplest, non-scented soap that suits you and that does not seem to cause or exacerbate any skin problems.

Do make sure, however, that you rinse thoroughly afterwards, using plenty of fresh, clean water. It is also important that you moisturise your skin properly. But I will deal with that a little later on.

Meanwhile, however, there are quite a few other aspects of skin cleansing which need to be dealt with.

There are, for example, the bubble baths and foam baths which are so much loved by film starlets and children. (Actually film starlets do not seem to bother so much about the bubbles these days – being pretty well prepared to pose without the need for any bubbles to protect their virtue.) Bubble and foam bath liquids contain surfactants, foam stabilizers and detergents and should not be used by anyone who suffers from eczema. These products do dry out the skin and cause all sorts of skin problems.

Nor should bath essences be used. There are many different types around but there is always a risk of producing a skin allergy reaction with these products. The only real point in using one of them is to make your bath smell nice and that is a fairly small advantage when you consider that the product could possibly make your eczema worse.

Bath oils, on the other hand, are much better. There are two main types: those which float on the surface of the water and those which disperse throughout the bath. These help by adding necessary oils to the skin.

Still in the general area of skin cleansing but moving away from soaps and bath additives we come to cleansing lotions, oils and creams.

Cleansing creams or cold creams consist of a mixture of olive oil, beeswax and water together with something like rosewater added to give fragrance. It is the evaporation of water from the mixture that makes the cream feel cool and gives it its name. The oil and wax in such a cream cleans the skin by loosening and picking up dirt and dead skin cells. In today's cleansing creams the olive oil is often replaced by mineral oil which is less likely to go 'off'. In addition to being of particular use for people whose skin is so dry and sensitive that they really cannot use soap, cleansing creams are useful for removing cosmetics from the skin.

Incidentally, cold creams used for cleansing used to be left on the skin as a moisturiser. This is no more logical than leaving a layer of dirty lather on the skin. Cleansing should always be considered an entirely separate act to moisturising.

If you do decide to use a cleansing cream, because you can not use soap or get your make up off properly with just soap, try to buy one that does not contain added fragrances, disinfectants or other additives. The thicker the cream, by the way, the more oil it contains while the thinner the cream the less oil and the more water. Cleansing milks are very 'thin' cold creams that contain a small amount of oil and a large amount of water.

This is probably a sensible place to point out, by the way, that cold creams and other cleansing creams are basically just the same as moisturising creams in that they are a mixture of oil and water. And you can, of course, use the same cream for both purposes. Vanishing creams, which have a high melting point and which are 'thin' in consistency get their name from the fact that when rubbed onto the skin they more or less disappear.

As cleansers, creams of this type help remove oils and oil products. As moisturisers these creams help cement the skin's rough surface layer of cells together, help to make the skin feel smoother and silkier and help prevent the loss of essential skin moisture. There are scores of different types of cream in this general category. All you have to do is find one which suits you.

When buying a skin cleansing cream, by the way, you can safely ignore the claims made by the cosmetic companies. Do not buy a cleansing lotion that contains any medicated ingredient, nor a cream designed to 'feed' or 'nourish' your skin at the same time (I will deal with nourishing creams more fully a little later on). By and large you are probably safest with one of the cheaper creams.

There is one other way that dirty skin can be cleaned and that is by using some sort of thinning or abrasive procedure. Dry skin often has a thick leathery outer layer with accumulated dead cells and blocked pores.

There are all sorts of suitable products that you can buy. There is for example the pumice stone: probably the oldest piece of bathroom hardware around and still as good as most modern aids for removing hard dry skin and superficial layers of dead cells. The pumice stone is made of volcanic lava. Alternatives include sea salt, which simply acts as an abrasive; the loofah, which is a dry, rough vegetable gourd; the friction mitt, which is a sort of synthetic loofah; and the ordinary bath brush. Or you can buy special products consisting of ground almonds, orange peel, strawberries or a fine oatmeal paste.

The simplest and cheapest product for thorough cleansing of dry skin is, however, probably the rough flannel. Just make sure that you have several and keep them clean.

Toning

The second traditional procedure in the skin care regime is toning.

This is a complete waste of time and money.

There are many, many different types of skin 'toner' around and as usual the cosmetics industry has dignified them with a series of important sounding names. There are astringents, fresheners and skin toners. One of the most important ingredients in all these products is alcohol which is there partly because when it evaporates it cools the skin (and therefore makes it feel 'fresh') and partly because it has a slightly irritating effect.

None of these so called skin toners has any lasting effect on your skin and you can probably get as useful an effect simply by patting cold water onto your skin with your bare hands.

Moisturising

In contrast to 'toning' the third traditional item in good skin care, moisturising, is vital.

Normally, skin contains a good deal of water. It is water that makes skin look fresh and healthy. Skin that has lost its natural moisture looks dry, wrinkled and cracked. It tends to feel uncomfortable. And it is likely to develop eczematous patches.

Because it is important to keep moisture levels as high as possible your skin produces a constant supply of natural oil, a substance designed to seal off the skin's surface and prevent the evaporation of those precious water supplies. Unfortunately, however, most of us remove that natural oil every time we wash. The oil disappears, together with the surface dirt and the dead skin cells. And the result is that without its natural oil the skin is left in a very vulnerable state. Water losses increase and the skin becomes dry and cracked.

It should be clear, therefore, that moisturising your skin is an important part of daily skin care. For eczema sufferers it is vital.

Moisturisers help enable us to replace those missing natural oils and to help keep the skin moist and fresh looking. Amazingly, many professional beauticians and so-called experts do not seem to understand this. They talk about moisturisers as though the creams were designed to add water to the skin. That is not true. Most moisturisers work by replacing lost oils and preventing the loss of moisture that is already there. Moisturisers work in much the same sort of way that waxed paper helps keep bread fresh – not by adding anything but by preserving what is already there.

Most of the moisturising creams on the market contain a mixture of two basic ingredients: oil and water. The thickness and texture and feel of the cream depends on just how much water and how much oil there is in the preparation. The thickest and most effective moisturiser will be one that contains a good deal of oil – a petroleum jelly would, for example, probably be as powerful a protective as you could possibly buy.

Although the basic constituents of a moisturising cream are simple, most manufacturers naturally do their very best to make their cream sound special. There are, therefore, those manufacturers who put shark oil, mink oil or avocado oil into their moisturisers. There is no advantage likely to be gained by buying one of these products. Nor will you gain anything from buying a moisturising cream which contains honey, seaweed, vitamin E, placenta extract or any of the other 'magical' ingredients that cosmetic companies are so fond of. The only thing such added ingredients will do is increase the price and the chances of you developing an allergy reaction.

The one ingredient manufacturers add which does have a powerful effect is the 'humectant'. Usually some substance such as glycerine, a humectant works by attracting moisture from the atmosphere. It could be described as the only genuine 'moisturising' cream in that it really does bring in moisture to the skin.

In theory the use of a humectant sounds rather attractive. In practice, however, there is one important problem. If there is not enough moisture in the atmosphere (and in many homes, shops and offices these days the atmosphere is very dry) then the humectant will have to attract water from somewhere else. And when lying on the skin the only other place it can get moisture from is the skin itself. So under these circumstances it can do more harm than good.

Because of this danger products containing humectants

should be avoided by eczema sufferers.

Moisturising is the single most important thing that eczema sufferers can do to protect their skin. You should buy several large pots of the cheapest moisturising cream that you can find which you both like and find acceptable. Then you should keep those pots scattered around the house – one in the bedroom, one in the bathroom and one in the kitchen.

You should always apply your moisturising cream after you have washed, remembering that if you put your cream on while the skin is slightly moist then your skin will be able to retain that extra moisture, and keep a jar near to the kitchen sink so that when you have been washing up you can apply some cream to your hands. Use a moisturising cream after a bath or shower and remember to put the cream all over your body – not forgetting your feet, elbows, arms and thighs. Those always seem to be areas that get forgotten.

Using a moisturiser regularly does not just help keep your skin moist, however. There are a couple of added bonuses. First, you will obtain some very real protection from the world around you. Very few of us live far away from factory chimneys these days and the air around us is often polluted, despite all the legislation that has been passed in recent years. You have only got to look at old buildings in city centres to see what damage the polluted atmosphere can do. Your moisturising cream will provide you with much needed protection against the acid in the air.

And a moisturising cream will, in addition, also protect you against the sun. Sunshine dries and ages the skin but the regular use of a moisturiser will help you avoid that particular problem.

Finally, there are the nourishing creams which are so popular among beauty editors. These are said to be able to feed your skin and to contain all sorts of essential ingredients. There are the products containing protein, vitamins and collagen, for example. The important thing to remember is that our skins cannot absorb foreign materials. The inner layers of the skin derive their nourishment from the blood supply they get and not from the outside world. The cells on the surface are dead and they need only water to remain healthy looking and plump and to give the skin a soft, smooth, appearance. In my view, there are no nourishing creams worth buying.

Skin care tips for eczema sufferers

● Use generous amounts of a simple, plain moisturising cream. Keep jars of your usual moisturiser spread around the house and use them regularly.

● Bath oils which disperse in the water and then adhere to your skin help to protect it.

● Do not over dry yourself after washing or bathing. If you leave your skin moist and then apply your moisturiser your skin will benefit.

● Do take special care to ensure that you always have a plentiful supply of fresh, clean towels – particularly in the kitchen. Although you should not rub your skin too hard, or over dry, it is important that you remove most of the moisture after washing.

● Make sure that you rinse your skin thoroughly after washing with soap or after having your hands in detergent. You should rinse with fresh, clean water.

● Be particularly careful to apply a moisturising cream to all parts of your skin that will be exposed when you are outside. In winter or summer a layer of moisturising cream will provide protection against pollutants in the atmosphere and against the sun.

● Do use cotton-lined rubber gloves when doing kitchen chores. Detergents, bleaches and other kitchen chemicals will damage your skin.

● Use a long-handled mop for cleaning dirty dishes. It will help you keep your hands out of the water as much as possible.

● Do not use bubble baths. They tend to have a drying effect on your skin.

● Take care not to let your home or office get too dry. Air conditioning frequently dries the air out. Turn down the air conditioning, open a window, buy a humidifier or make sure that there are bowls of water standing near to the radiators.

● Do not lie in the bath for more than twenty minutes. Showers are better for you than baths. Do not bathe in water that is uncomfortably hot.

- If you go swimming in public baths make sure that you rinse yourself thoroughly afterwards. The chlorine in the water is bad for your skin.
- Wear gloves in the winter to protect your hands from the cold weather.
- Try to drink several glasses of fresh water each day. If your intake of fluid is too low your body is bound to be deprived of essential moisture.
- Protect yourself against the sun by wearing a wide brimmed floppy hat in the summer and by using sun-screening agents.

Eczema and your nails

If the skin around your nails is affected by eczema then the eczema may affect your nails too and they will become ridged or broken. You should ideally treat your nails and the area around them in just the same way as any other patch of eczema. Do remember, however, that fungal infections of the nails are quite common and so any nail problem which persists merits a visit to your doctor.

Adapt your personality

Earlier (see pages 11-14) I explained just how your personality can affect your chances of developing eczema. There are many other factors which decide whether or not you are going to develop eczema but 'personality' is undoubtedly a critical one. And even though I do not pretend for an instant that you can change your personality (nor do I think it would be a good idea to try) you can certainly *adapt* your personality and your way of life in such a way that your skin will benefit.

LET YOUR EMOTIONS OUT

Do not store up tears inside you. There is now evidence to show that when we cry there are very good reasons for it. Not only does our crying make it clear to those around us that we need extra comfort and attention, but the tears we shed contain harmful substances that our bodies need to get rid of when we are upset. The research work in this area is still in its infancy but it does seem likely that if you refuse to cry your body will store up harmful chemicals and you will end up with a genuine, fully blown depression.

I am not suggesting that you open the floodgates at every possible opportunity. But do not be afraid to cry in front of those who are close to you, or in private. Store up the tears and you will probably make your eczema worse. Let the tears out and you will probably help your eczema.

Similarly, just as it is unwise to store up tears and sadness so it is unwise to store up anger and aggression. If you feel really cross about something and you say and do nothing about it then your body will be storing up a great deal of repressed anger. And that can be dangerous. It can, for example, induce an attack of eczema.

You do not have to shout at everyone who annoys you, or hit people who make you cross. That would not help much. But you should learn to get rid of your anger and aggression in other ways: perhaps by smashing a ball on a golf course or squash court, or by beating a carpet in the garden, or doing some digging, or smashing some old plates in the garage, or even by investing in, and using, a punchball.

LEARN THAT YOU CAN BE HAPPY AND HEALTHY

If you were brought up to associate affection and love with your skin condition then you are probably going to find it difficult to break free of those constraints. Just by understanding the problem, however, you can do a great deal to help yourself.

Parents should remember too that it is extremely important not to encourage children to grow up associating affection with poor health.

DEAL WITH YOUR STRESS

Many people who suffer from stress fear that in order to cope with it they will have to take up something rather odd – join a religious sect or start wrapping their legs around their heads, for example. The fact is, however, that in order to relax you do not have to do anything strange. All you have to do is read the advice given later in this section. (See pages 62-67.)

COPE WITH YOUR GUILT

First of all you must, of course, decide whether or not any particular feeling of guilt is really justified or not. Obviously, if you are feeling guilty because of something that you have done (run into a parked car or broken a cup for example) then the only solution is to apologise and make what amends you can. In most instances, however, guilt is far more complex than that. If you are the sort of individual who tends to suffer from guilt then you probably feel guilty because of things you have not done and because of your own suspicions about how other people will feel and respond.

This is the type of guilt that causes most pain and to deal with it you must first of all find out exactly why it is you feel guilty. Is it because you feel that you have failed someone such as your mother, your employer, your spouse or your God? Much of the guilt we suffer is produced by our relationships with those who are very close to us (love is the greatest single cause of guilt) and so in order to protect yourself you must learn to differentiate between the realistic expectations of those who are close to you and their unrealistic demands. You must learn not to allow other people to put those sorts of demands on you or your conscience.

So, for example, you should perhaps not feel guilty if you can not visit your parents every week, if you cannot buy your children all the toys they want, if you cannot do all the overtime that your employer would like you to do, and so on.

The truth about individuals who suffer a lot from guilt is they tend to be thoughtful and caring people.

If you suffer a lot from pangs of guilt it is probably because you care too much about other people; you probably worry too much about what other people think, about what other people feel and about how your actions are going to be seen.

I know that this may sound strange but to protect yourself a little and to keep your skin in good condition you need to be a little more selfish, a little more self aware and a little more able to appreciate your own very good points. If you are the sort of individual who is driven by guilt then you are probably conscientious, hard working, ambitious, thoughtful, reliable, honest and generous. Despite all these good points you probably think of yourself as a failure and you are probably far too critical about what you do. You probably expect far more from yourself than you would ever dream of expecting from anyone else – and some of the people around you may well take advantage of this trait.

I suggest that you sit yourself down and write down a list of all your good points. Pretend that you are writing your own obituary and be honest and fair with yourself. You will almost certainly end up with a fairly long list of good things that you could say about yourself. Now, being equally honest and impartial, try to list all your bad points. Look for things that you would criticise in other people. I bet your list of bad points is much shorter than your list of good points.

Next time you are swamped with guilt take a look at your two lists, take a little pride in yourself and learn to be a little more selfish. Your eczema will benefit enormously.

CONTROL YOUR FEARS
Fear can be debilitating, and can have a bad effect on your skin. To cope with your fears you must recognise and face those things that worry you most. The unknown, unidentified fear is much more dangerous and more damaging than the fear that has been carefully examined.

Once you have made a list of all the things that really worry you then you can go through the list and see what you can do to help yourself worry less. So, for example, if you worry a good deal about your health it may be wise to visit your family doctor for a complete check up. Or better still, make a positive decision to learn more about your body and to come to terms with just what you need to do in order to conquer your problems. Self awareness and understanding will last much longer in your battle against fear than professional reassurance, necessary as it is.

If your fears concern money or employment the same is true. Once you have made a very precise list of all the things that worry you then you are much more likely to be able to do something to help yourself. You will not be able to solve all your fears or eradicate all your worries straight away, of course. But you will be able to do something to help yourself. And that always makes a tremendous difference to the way that your body – and your skin – responds.

Learn to relax your body

Stress and eczema are closely linked. If you learn how to relax your muscles, and your body, then you can not only get rid of some of your anxiety but you may also be able to improve the condition of your skin.

To relax your muscles you must first learn just how your muscles feel when they are tight and tense. To start with, clench your fist. As you do you will feel the muscles of your hand and forearm tighten and become firm. Now, gradually let your fist unfold. This time you will feel the muscles slowly relax. To relax your muscles, all you have to do is to stiffen and then relax them group by group.

When you first start relaxing you should choose a quiet, private place where you are not likely to be interrupted and where stimuli are least disturbing. It is difficult to relax in a crowded department store or on a busy train – although you will probably be able to do that eventually.

Start by lying down in a darkened room where you are likely to be left alone for at least a quarter of an hour – you should allow a quarter of an hour for each session to start with and you will need to plan on spending that much time every day for a week or so until you have mastered the art of physical relaxation.

Here is the step-by-step programme for physical relaxation.

1 Clench your left hand as firmly as you can, making a fist of your fingers. Clench it hard and you will see your knuckles turning white. Then gradually let your fist unfold and as you do so you will feel the muscles relax.

2 Bend your left arm so that your left biceps muscle stands out. Then relax and let the muscles ease. Let your arm lie loosely by your side and try to ignore it.

3 Relax your right hand in exactly the same way.

4 Relax your right biceps muscle in the same way.

5 Tighten the muscles in your left foot. Curl your toes. When the foot feels as tense as you can make it, let it relax.

6 Tense the muscles of your left calf. If you reach down you can feel the muscles at the back of your leg firm up as you tense them. Bend your foot back at the ankle to help tighten up the muscles. Then let the muscles relax.

7 Straighten your leg and push your foot away from you. You will feel the muscles on the front of your thigh tighten up; they should be firm right up to the top of your leg. Then let the muscles relax.

8 Tense and relax your right foot.

9 Tense and relax your right lower leg.

10 Tense and relax your right thigh.

11 Lift yourself up by tightening up your buttock muscles. You will be able to lift your body upwards by an inch or so. Then let the muscles fall loose again.

12 Tense and contract your abdominal muscles. Try to pull your abdominal wall as far in as possible. Then let go and allow your waist to reach its maximum circumference.

13 Tighten the muscles of your chest. Take a big, deep breath and strain to hold it for as long as possible. Then let go.

14 Push your shoulders backwards as far as they will go, then turn them forwards and inwards. Finally, shrug them as high as you can. Keep your head perfectly still and try to touch your ears with your shoulders. It will probably be impossible but try it anyway. Then let your shoulders relax and ease.

15 Next, tighten up the muscles of your back. Try to make yourself as tall as you possibly can. Then let the muscles relax.

16 The muscles of your neck are next. Lift your head forward and pull at the muscles at the back of your neck. Turn your head first one way and then the other way. Push your head backwards with as much force as you can. Then let the muscles of your neck relax. Move it about to make sure that it really is loose and easy.

17 Move your eyebrows upwards and then pull them down as far as they will go. Do this several times, making sure that you can feel the muscles tightening both when you move the eyebrows up and when you pull them down again. Then let them relax.

18 Screw up your eyes as tightly as you can. Pretend that someone is trying to force your eyes open. Keep them shut tightly. Then, keeping your eyelids closed let them relax.

19 Move your lower jaw around. Grit your teeth. Wrinkle your nose. Smile as wide as you can, showing as many teeth as you have got. Now let all those facial muscles relax.

20 Push your tongue out as far as it will go, push it firmly against the bottom of your mouth and the top of your mouth and then let it lie relaxed and easy inside your mouth.

As you do all these simple exercises remember that your breathing should be slow, deep and regular. Take deep breaths and breathe as slowly as you comfortably can.

You will probably begin to feel calmer and more relaxed after just one session of physical relaxation. But remember that you really need to persist with this physical relaxation programme. As you become more experienced you will not have to relax step-by-step but will be able to relax your whole body more or less instantly.

Learn to relax your mind

One of the easiest and most effective ways to deal with stress and to stop anxiety, fear and worry affecting your skin is to learn how to relax your mind. There is now evidence from all parts of the world to show that patients can improve their health and well being a tremendous amount by learning how to relax their minds.

Under normal, everyday circumstances an unending stream of facts and feelings pour into your mind. Even when you are not consciously 'thinking' or 'worrying', your eyes, nose, ears and other sense organs will be pushing thousands of bits and pieces of unwanted information into your mind. Together, all these pieces of information help to produce stress and pressure. If you can cut the number of messages going into your brain then you will be able to ease the amount of stress on your mind. And the effect on your skin will almost certainly be beneficial. It certainly won't be harmful!

Many of the people who recommend mental relaxation suggest that you should try to empty your mind completely in order to cut out the damaging effect of all this information.

The problem is, of course, that trying to empty your mind of all the conscious and subconscious messages that keep streaming into it is not easy. Indeed, very many people find the prospect of emptying their minds completely so terrifying that they never even try. And so they lose the possibility of benefiting from simple mental relaxation.

Fortunately, however there is another way to cut down the amount of damaging information pouring into your mind. And that is to fill your mind with pleasant, peaceful, relaxing thoughts. In other words, all that you have to do is to re-learn how to daydream. I say 're-learn' deliberately because you will almost certainly have been able to daydream when you were small. But you were probably taught (by both your parents and your teachers) that daydreaming is wasteful and rather naughty.

Incidentally, it should be clear from this that I recommend that parents with children suffering from eczema allow their offspring to daydream from time to time. (See page 68.)

Daydreaming works for several reasons. First, it works because your body will respond to an imagined world just as effectively as it will respond to the real world. When the film *Lawrence of Arabia* was shown in the cinema a few years ago, cinema managers around the world were astonished to find that the sales of cold drinks and ice creams rocketed. Even when the heating failed in one particular cinema and the temperature plummeted the patrons still wanted to buy cold drinks and ice creams. The explanation was that the cinema patrons were responding to the desert scenes that they were watching on the screen. Their bodies responded as though the desert was entirely real. So, fill your mind with some pleasant, relaxing, imaginery scene and your body will respond as though the scene were real. The horrors of the real world around you will be forgotten.

The second reason why daydreaming works so well is that the human body responds positively to good, happy, feelings. When we are frightened or worried we respond badly: we feel upset, we get indigestion and headaches and our skin condition may get worse. But when we are happy and contented there is a very clear and useful healing effect on the body. So, if you learn how to daydream you will benefit in both those ways.

And your skin will very probably benefit too.

When you begin re-learning how to daydream you will probably have to find somewhere quiet and peaceful. You will need to be able to cut out the world. Later on, when you have mastered the art, you will be able to do it just about anywhere.

So, to start with, lie yourself down on your bed, close the door, take the telephone off the hook, feed the animals and draw the curtains. Put a 'Do Not Disturb' notice on the door.

Once you are peacefully settled try to remember some particularly happy and peaceful scene from your past. It is best to use a real scene because you will be better able to re-create all the necessary feelings. But you can, if you like, use an entirely fictional scene.

If you are using a scene from your past then you might try a beach scene from a good holiday by the sea. With your eyes firmly closed take big, deep breaths as slowly and as regularly as you possibly can. And then slowly try to feel the warmth of the sun on your face. Try not to let anyone else into your daydream by the way. If you let people into your daydream then you are likely either to end up with a nightmare or with a fantasy. And neither is likely to be particularly relaxing.

Once you can feel the sun on your face try to imagine that you can hear the sound of the waves breaking on the shore. And try to feel the warm, soft sand underneath you. Listen to the seagulls circling overhead and smell the salty sea air. Allow a gentle breeze to play over your body.

Once your mind has been convinced then your body will be

convinced too. The accumulated pressures from the real world will slowly disappear. As your mind is filled with all these peaceful thoughts so your body will begin to respond. And eventually your skin will benefit.

You do not, of course, have to restrict yourself to this one particular daydream. You can build up your very own, personal library of useful daydreams. There can be real memories, there can be fictional memories, and there can be memories taken from films or books. It does not matter what the memory is as long as the effect is to make you feel happy and peaceful, and as long as you can create memories that are convincing.

Reduce your stress by organising your life

The motorist who remembers to buy petrol for his car and put air into the tyres will be far less likely to find himself stressed by running out of fuel or having a 'blow out' on the motorway. The shopper who knows in advance what he is going to buy will be far less likely to end up making a second trip to the shops. The businessman who plans ahead will be less likely to end up with a crisis on his hands. Bad organisation and poor planning will often lead to anxiety, increased stress loads and exacerbated eczema. Learn to organise your life and you will reduce the number of crises which might make your eczema worse.

Follow this simple four-stage plan.

1   Keep a diary that contains details of all events that need advance planning (birthdays, anniversaries etc). Get into the habit of examining it each morning to make sure that you know just what you have to do. Advance planning for trips and meetings of all kinds obviously helps to reduce the risk of something going wrong.

2   Keep an efficient filing system to enable you to store bills, letters and receipts just where you can find them. There is nothing more frustrating than hunting around for an important letter and wasting hours on the job. You do not have to buy a filing cabinet – you can use old brown envelopes or a cardboard box.

3 When you have got a really difficult problem to solve do not let it ruin your life — simply write down all the possible solutions in a notebook. Keep the list somewhere safe and near to you and add new solutions as they occur to you. Keep the list by you when you are in the bath, in the car or in bed: those are the places where ideas tend to come to you. Then, when you finally need to make a decision take a look down your list of possibilities and you will probably find that one particular answer stands out. You will certainly be able to cross out many of the alternatives which seemed logical when you wrote them down but which by now look silly.

4 Keep a notebook and pencil with you at all times. Jot down any thought that needs remembering or needs action. When they are put down on paper problems always seem slightly less significant. And you will not have to worry about remembering them either.

Protect your children from stress

Children are just as susceptible to stress and pressure as adults. Something like one half of all childhood illnesses and ailments are either produced by or exacerbated by stress. Eczema is one of the diseases known to be most affected.

It is clearly important, therefore, that all parents with children suffering from eczema know how to ensure that their children are not exposed to too much stress.

The advice which follows should help.

● Do not always expect your child to be doing something useful. Many parents tell their children off if they find them day-dreaming but it is a simple and natural way of relaxing. There is nothing wrong with your child escaping from the real world into a daydream every now and again. The only time to get worried is if he never seems to come back to reality.

● Do try and spend some time each day talking to your child, finding out what sort of things are worrying him and encouraging him to share his problems with you.

● Do not let your child get involved in too many high pressure activities. Encourage him to spend some time relaxing on things that do not really matter very much. We live in a very high pressure society today and children of all ages are encouraged to do well in many different areas. By the time they reach the age of six or seven many children are already under pressure to do well at school.

There are even many parents and teachers who put their children under pressure to do well on the sports fields and in the athletics arena. There are cups to be won, prizes to be collected and trophies to be accumulated. I have seen toddlers crying because their team has been beaten and I have met children with hands blistered by hours of practice with golf club or tennis racket.

● Many children are put under pressure by various forms of manipulation. As parents we are skilled at getting our children to do what we want them to do by making them feel guilty. When you say 'you wouldn't do that if you loved me', 'if only you knew what sacrifices we've made for you', 'you're making your mother ill' or 'I don't know what we've done to deserve this sort of treatment' you are manipulating your child by using guilt as a weapon. You may not be particularly conscious of attempting to force your child to behave in a certain way but unconsciously you are doing just that. Guilt is an extremely powerful weapon and is especially dangerous when allowed to intrude into a relationship based largely on love and natural affection.

The more sensitive your child is the more likely he is to be put under pressure and stress by such simple, manipulative phrases. And gentle, emotional blackmail of this kind produces more long lasting and damaging stress than shouting, screaming, threatening or even beating your child.

● Do not put too much pressure on your child to grow up. Many children are struggling to cope with the physical, mental and emotional problems of puberty while at the same time being expected to cope with some of the responsibilities normally shouldered by adults.

I have met children who have been expected to do the family shopping and housework, children who have been making their own meals at the age of ten and children who have been expected to act as interpreters and translators for entire

69

families. Often children with one parent will be expected to provide support, advice and comfort in place of the missing spouse.

Try to let your child enjoy his childhood. He will not get another chance.

● Children do adapt to change very well. Even quite small children quickly become accustomed to the fact that there are few stable factors in the world around them. Buildings are knocked down, pop singers come in and out of fashion, clothes that are 'with it' one month can be quite out of date a few weeks later.

Nevertheless, there are some aspects of modern life that even children may find daunting. By the time he is old enough to vote your child may have watched something like one hundred thousand television commercials, seen thousands of newspaper and magazine advertisements and been exposed to advertising propaganda while in the cinemas and while listening to the radio.

It is hardly surprising that, under these continuing pressures, many children grow up with entirely artificial tastes and needs; tastes and needs that have been designed and nurtured by an unseen army of hidden manipulators.

You may be able to help your child cope with this deluge of commercially inspired misinformation by teaching him a little scepticism and cynicism.

● Remember that the television set can be a potential source of stress. Children these days love the 'box' so much that when a group of four-to-six-year-olds were recently asked which they liked best, television or daddy, nearly half said that they preferred TV. That is frightening. Particularly since the television set is commonly used as a permanently available electronic babysitter. The percentage who prefer TV will probably increase in the future.

It is frightening because it is now a recognised fact that many children have nightmares as a direct result of watching frightening films on television. A recent survey showed that one in three school children dream about programmes that they have watched. When you realise that a TV diet consists largely of murders, rapes and miscellaneous acts of butchery it is hardly surprising that children's viewing habits often lead to nightmares and stress.

If you have a child who suffers from eczema remember these points. Obviously not all childhood eczema is caused by stress. But all cases of childhood eczema will be made worse by stress.

Protect yourself at work

If your eczema seems to be related to your job then there are a number of things that you can do to help yourself.

● Always make sure that you wash and rinse yourself very well after work. Make sure that you use plenty of fresh water. Use soap too if there is oil to remove. If possible wash your hands after every contact with possible irritants – but if you do this then do also make sure that you dry your hands thoroughly afterwards and then re-apply your normal moisturising cream. If your whole body comes into contact with some possible irritant then you should wash all of it thoroughly as soon as possible.

● Use a base cream or barrier cream on all those areas of your skin that could possibly be exposed to the irritant. You should use a barrier cream even if you also wear protective clothing.

● Protective clothing is useful and important. If you wear rubber gloves make sure that they are cotton-lined. If you are given special overalls to wear then make sure that you wear them. They will not do you much good hanging up in your locker.

● Use whatever aids are available. Do not, for example, put your hands into an irritant liquid if there is a pick up stick or probe that you can use instead.

● Always make sure that you keep your doctor fully informed about your work. If you are an eczema sufferer then your doctor should have a record of your job. Your doctor may know of problems associated with it and he may be able to offer you special advice.

● If your eczema persists despite all your efforts to deal with it, and you know that your eczema is caused by your work then you have to make a simple but important decision: whether to carry on with your job and put up with the skin problem, or to look for something safer to give your skin a chance to recover. No one but you can possibly make this decision.

Protect your skin against the sun

Lying on the beach acquiring a suntan may be fashionable but it is not sensible.

The sun damages the skin more effectively than any other single external factor. If, despite this warning, you still feel inclined to risk all and expose yourself to the sun, then you should do so with caution and a little preparation. As an eczema sufferer you have more to lose than anyone else. Apart from being partly responsible for the ageing process that causes wrinkling of the skin, sunshine also produces dryness and will exacerbate any existing skin problem such as eczema.

There are, of course, a great many ways in which you can protect yourself from the sun.

The most obvious way is to keep out of the sun when it is at its most dangerous. This may sound very obvious but it is always surprising just how many tourists and holiday-makers forget that the sun is much hotter and more dangerous at mid-day. While the locals keep to the shade, and sip cool drinks, the tourists will be out there with Noel Coward's mad dogs, mopping their brows and watching their skin peel away.

If you cannot keep out of the sun there are many ways in which you can protect yourself. Read through the following notes and follow whichever pieces of advice seem appropriate.

● Your choice of clothes can have a dramatic effect on your skin. A broad brimmed hat is one of the most obvious ways of obtaining protection and those Mexican bandits did not wear them because they looked quaintly romantic. Long sleeved, loose fitting cotton clothes also provide protection. Sunshades and sun umbrellas may be slightly old fashioned but they do provide shade.

Remember too that you can be affected by the sun while swimming. If your skin is becoming dry you may need to wear an old cotton shirt while bathing.

● If you have fair or red hair and light blue eyes then you are likely to burn very easily and you are also more likely to develop skin problems if you spend a lot of time in the sun.

● Sand, water, snow and white buildings all reflect the sun's rays and can increase the speed at which your skin suffers.

● Remember that you do not have to be sunbathing for your skin to be affected by the sun. Even while playing games such as tennis your skin can be burnt.

● If you intend to expose parts of your body that do not normally get exposed (if you are going topless for example) then do be particularly careful. Such delicate areas as nipples can become very sore if exposed to too much sunshine.

● Creams and lotions designed to give you an artificial tan are probably harmless enough in themselves but do not be tempted into thinking that because you have got a false tan then you can still go out into the sun without getting burnt. It is not true. You can burn just as easily as if you did not have the tan at all.

● Do not sunbathe while wearing perfume. You may develop blotchy patches on your skin. And those blotches can sometimes be permanent.

● Do be particularly careful if you are taking prescribed drugs and you go out into the sun. Blotchiness can develop and may be permanent with drugs too. Antibiotics, contraceptives, diuretics and tranquillisers have all been shown to cause this particular problem. Check with your doctor if you are taking a prescribed drug and plan to go out in the sun a good deal.

● Creams and lotions will provide you with your most important protection. Ordinary moisturising creams are probably the simplest, cheapest and easiest to use. The thinner the cream the less the protection you will get. If you choose a cold cream, however, you will get quite a lot of useful protection. The important thing to remember when using a moisturising cream is that you have to use liberal quantities and you have to apply the cream regularly. Do remember that all creams are easily washed or wiped off when you are bathing or lying on a towel.

It is vitally important, too, to remember that your protective cream must be applied to every piece of skin which may be exposed. Do not just plaster the moisturiser onto those areas of skin which most commonly develop eczematous patches. Do not forget your neck and lips, for example. And do not forget your shoulders and ankles. The parts of your body where the bone is nearest to the surface (and where, therefore, the skin is thinnest) are the most vulnerable.

Although simple moisturising creams are useful, in that they do not simply keep the sun's rays away from your skin but also prevent too much drying out, the most effective products to buy to protect your skin are creams which contain a proper sunscreening agent. These products will help you acquire a tan without your skin being too adversely affected by the sun. As with so many other cosmetic products the main problem here is differentiating between the rival claims made by different companies.

If you want something to keep the sun's rays away from the skin almost entirely then you need a total sunscreen. The best products in this category usually contain something like zinc oxide. Known as sun barrier creams these products do not let any sun through at all and they are most useful for individuals who have very dry or sensitive skin and who want to go out into the sunshine but who are frightened of the effect it may have on their skin.

Most people, however, do not really want to keep all the sun's rays off their skin. They want some protection but they also want to acquire a slight tan. This yearning for the best of both worlds is not entirely impractical, for there are some useful creams around which provide protection while letting you get a tan.

Chemicals which filter out the shorter length rays include para-aminobenzoic acid, the benzphenone derivatives and a number of other substances. These compounds vary in their efficiency, their tendency to stain clothes, their likelihood of irritating the skin and their ability to stay on the skin when it is wet. To choose an effective sunscreen you have to rely on the scale used by manufacturers to grade their products. And then you have to experiment with the various available products until you manage to find one that suits you.

Most manufacturers give their products 'delay factors' and print this information on the box or package or the tube. The theory is that if you pick a cream with a delay factor of six then that cream will delay burning for six times as long as usual.

Unfortunately, there is no generally accepted scale for these delay factors and manufacturers can largely decide for themselves what number they give their product. However, this is the only system there is so I am afraid you will have to make the best of it.

If you have very sensitive or normally dry skin then I suggest you look for a cream with a delay factor of at least ten to fourteen.

These simple sunscreen products are effective and useful. They provide some protection and enable people with dry skin or with disorders such as eczema to enjoy their summer holidays. However, there are a number of manufacturers now enthusiastically offering sunscreen products which also contain an accelerator. The theory here is that the sunscreen protects your skin while the accelerator helps you get a tan as quickly as possible. These accelerators seem to work by increasing the sensitivity of the skin to the types of ultraviolet light which produce tanning.

If you have dry or sensitive skin, or you suffer from eczema then I do not recommend these products. I'm not convinced that they are entirely safe or that they are worth the extra money you will have to pay for them.

As a general rule the most important thing to remember when choosing a cream is to choose something that you can buy cheaply. If it is cheap you will be able to buy fairly large quantities of it, and you will not mind applying the cream liberally. With sunscreen creams it is the amount you use as much as the content of the cream that determines the quality of the protection you get.

Finally, even if you have black skin, or very well sun-tanned skin, do remember that you must use a moisturing cream to protect your skin against dryness.

Irritant or allergic eczema: finding the cause

If you suffer from eczema and you suspect that you have irritant or allergic eczema then look through the list that follows to see if you can find a possible cause.

• If your eczema affects your whole body.

Your skin problem is most likely to be due to an allergen that has been swallowed. Foods or drugs are the most likely explanation. Remember that the skin sometimes takes about ten days to respond to internal allergens.

• If the eczema is around your mouth.

Saliva is the most likely cause. But medicines, sweets, cosmetics and toothpaste are also possible explanations.

• If the eczema is confined to your scalp.

Think about shampoos, conditioners, hair dyes, hair colourants and so on. All these are possible causes of skin symptoms on the scalp.

• If your eczema is confined to your ears.

Then spectacle frames, ear rings, ear studs and hearing aids are all possible villains.

• If your eczema is confined to the area around your eyes and nose.

Put cosmetics and skin creams at the top of your list.

• If your eczema is confined to your feet.

Shoes, socks and foot powders are the most likely causes of your problem.

• If your eczema is confined to your hands and arms.

Then look at rings, watch straps, bracelets, soaps, shirt cuffs and jumper sleeves. Remember that the wrists may be the only part of your body to come into constant contact with a woolly jumper – or with the soap powder that the jumper was washed in. Remember too that you may wash your hands in several different types of soap during the day.

• If your eczema is confined to your trunk or body.

Clothes are the most likely explanation. Belts, buckles, zips, press studs and other fasteners are likely to produce localised reactions. But jumpers, shirts and underclothes may produce larger rashes. As may washing powders. It is important to rinse clothes thoroughly even when non-biological washing powders are used. Do not forget that clothes bought as Christmas or birthday gifts may produce rashes if they are made of material which you do not normally wear.

Finally, you should be aware that up to one third of all cases of contact eczema are caused or complicated by skin creams and ointments which have either been prescribed by a doctor or bought over a chemist's counter. You should think of this possibility if your eczema seems to be getting worse during treatment or if it does not seem to be getting any better.

Avoiding allergies

I doubt if there is any substance in the world to which someone, somewhere has not developed an allergy rash.

At Christmas, for example, thousands of unhappy people develop rashes to the presents they have been given. Deodorants, perfumes, hair sprays, aftershaves, and so on all cause nasty red, raw rashes. So do some clothes, of course. And there are many, many individuals who are allergic to different types of metal and who develop rashes when they try wearing new rings, brooches, necklaces and bracelets. (Incidentally, if you do have an allergy rash to a piece of jewellery but you want to continue to wear it, then try painting it with clear nail varnish.)

Washing powders, particularly some of the more powerful 'biological' powders, cause a lot of trouble too. As do tanning lotions, sun-tan creams, artificial tans and medicated soaps. Even some creams and ointments sold to relieve skin problems can cause allergy problems of their own.

It is important too to remember that although many allergy reactions do develop quite soon after contact with the irritant it is possible for there to be a long delay between the contact and the development of the rash. And you may develop an allergy to something that you have been using, apparently safely, for many years.

Remember too, that you do not have to have been in contact with a large amount of an allergen to acquire a problem. You can react badly to a small amount of a chemical. And do not forget that allergens can often get onto your skin in all sorts of indirect ways. So, for example, nail varnish can cause an allergy reaction on the face if you touch your face with your nails. And a woman wearing lipstick can produce an allergy rash on the face of a man she kisses. I am afraid that the permutations for distress are endless.

There are a number of things that you can do, however, to reduce your risk of developing a skin allergy.

● You can patch test yourself when buying or starting to use any new product. (See below.)
● Stick to products that you know are safe. When one major washing powder manufacturer recently changed a leading powder there were thousands of complaints from users who claimed that they had developed problems when using the new version. The manufacturers then relented and put the old product back on sale.
● Try to buy hypo-allergenic products whenever possible. Some companies claim to make non-allergenic products but that is nonsense. There is nothing in the world that can be described as entirely safe. Hypo-allergenic products are simply products that are less likely to cause problems because they contain only ingredients which are known to be unlikely to cause rashes.
● If you have sensitive skin be particularly careful with depilatories (chemicals for removing unwanted hair), hair wave lotions and hair straighteners, bleaches of all kinds, nail enamels, hair colourants and perfumes. These are all known to be common causes of allergy problems.
● Remember, that once you have acquired an allergy to a particular substance you are likely to retain that allergy. You can try the product again after a couple of years if you really want to – but generally speaking once you have an allergy you have got it for life.

Patch testing

If your eczema is caused or made worse by an allergy to one substance or a series of substances you should be careful when applying anything new to your skin. This means taking care with new cosmetics, hair dyes, hair colourants, bleaches and hair removing creams.

The best way of protecting yourself is to test a small amount of any new substance on one area of skin, rather than going ahead and using large quantities of what may prove to be an uncomfortable and annoying irritant.

This is known as 'patch testing'.

To do this simply impregnate a small piece of gauze with the substance that you are trying out, fix it to your skin with a small piece of sticking plaster (make sure that you use sticking plaster that you know does not cause you any problems) and leave it in position for forty-eight hours.

It does not matter where you stick it as long as it is somewhere where you can examine the result easily afterwards. And it is better to put your test patch on an area that is not going to be visible or cause much discomfort.

If, when you remove the plaster, you find that you have developed an itchy, blotchy red rash then you would be well advised to give the rest of the test substance away to someone else. If it is perfume that you have been trying you could try putting it onto your clothes instead of your skin.

Incidentally, when buying new products from shops ask if you can patch test yourself in the shop. This will save you the unnecessary expense of investing in a product that you will not be able to use.

Avoiding common irritants and allergens

Although it is possible for the skin to be irritated by an enormous number of different substances there are a small number of particularly troublesome irritants and allergens that you should try to avoid.

NICKEL

Nickel is one of the commonest causes of eczema. It is present in kitchen utensils, scissors, sewing needles, thimbles, many household appliances, silver coins, pen-knives, pens, lighters, keys, bag fittings, metal parts on umbrellas, foreign silver and gold, jewellery clasps, ear-rings and bracelets, bra fastenings, metal buttons, studs, zips and suspenders. If it is not possible to replace nickel items then they can usually be covered with tape or with lacquer (or with clear nail varnish).

RUBBER

There are troublesome rubbers in some oils and sprays as well as in rubber gloves (it is because the rubber may cause an allergy reaction that it is particularly important to wear cotton glove liners inside rubber gloves) and corsets. Rubber grips on household appliances and on bicycles may also cause problems.

LANOLIN
Widely used in cosmetics and some handcreams, lanolin can cause all sorts of skin troubles.

FRAGRANCES
Perfumes themselves can cause skin irritation but many other substances also contain added fragrances which can cause irritation. You should, therefore, take care with handcreams (including moisturisers), soaps, cleansers, polishes, sprays, spices, herbs and many other household items.

Other items you should be especially careful of are:
Sticking plaster, dyes, detergents, plants, anti-histamine creams, golf club and tennis racket handles and, sadly, pets.

Itching without scratching

Eczematous patches can be terribly itchy and it can be almost impossible not to seek relief by scratching. Unfortunately, since patches of eczema tend to be raw and open it is easy for them to get infected. And infected patches of eczema are even more un-sightly, more uncomfortable and more difficult to deal with than uninfected patches.

So it is important to scratch as little as possible. There are several ways of seeking relief without scratching.

● Try not to stay too close to hot fires or radiators. And try not to have the central heating turned up too high. You are more likely to itch if you feel hot.
● Try to wear cotton clothes – they are cooler and less likely to cause itching than wool.
● Use a cool, soothing cream to stop itching. Bland, plain creams can be used quite liberally without danger.
●A splash of cold water will often ease itching.

- Anti-histamine tablets will stop itching. Unfortunately, they tend to cause drowsiness and so are best kept for night-time itching.

Creams and ointments you can buy yourself

Many different companies make products which are sold as cures or treatments for eczema.

There are creams available containing just about every conceivable ingredient: animal, vegetable or mineral.

The only creams worth buying not on a prescription are simple, plain moisturising creams. Find a cream that suits your skin, that is cheap and use it generously.

Evening primrose oil

In the last few years evening primrose oil has gained something of a reputation as a magical 'cure-all'. It has been recommended for many different disorders and has proved particularly popular among those searching for cures for premenstrual tension and for eczema.

The evening primrose is a wild flower and the oil is obtained from the seeds. The first modern research to show that evening primrose oil had a beneficial effect on eczema was done in 1981. It showed that when taken in capsule form the oil produced a thirty per cent improvement in the severity of symptoms.

Since then other trials have been started but not yet completed. It does seem that the oil is safe although some patients, for example those with temporal lobe epilepsy, should not take it. It will probably be some time before there is any conclusive evidence one way or the other. Since it does *seem* to be free of side effects I can see no harm in patients conducting their own trials if other methods of control do fail. Capsules containing 500 mg of evening primrose oil are obtainable from many pharmacies. You should adjust your dosage according to the manufacturer's recommendations and I suggest strongly that you have a word with your doctor before you begin the course.

Alternative practitioners – a word of warning

Disillusioned with the medical care offered by orthodox medical practitioners, thousands of people are these days turning to the many different alternative therapies that are now available.

Some forms of alternative medicine do work. And many practitioners in this field are reliable, honest and trustworthy. But there are several general points which must be made.

● There are very few laws and regulations governing what can be done by (and claimed for) alternative practitioners. There are, I am afraid, a number of quacks and charlatans around whose main aim is to part you from your money. They will play on your fears and aspirations in order to do this. Unless proper state registration is introduced for all forms of alternative medicine this problem is likely to remain.

Alternative practitioners sometimes claim that their remedies are without risk. But this assertion is misleading. For instance, some herbal remedies, which are often described as being without risk, contain powerful constituents which can be dangerous. Acupuncturists who do not sterilize their needles properly can pass on hepatitis. Hypnotherapists who practice regression can trigger off severe mental problems.

● Remember that the placebo response has a powerful effect on all types of medical treatment. If you believe that something is going to work, and you want it to work, the chances are high that it will work. Researchers have shown that if one hundred people are given sugar pills to treat their pain then between a third and a half of them will get considerable relief. When the sugar pill is given with enthusiasm then the chances of it working are that much greater. We know now that the placebo response relies on the body's own internal hormone production – and that there are, for example, pain relieving hormones available within the body. There is no doubt that some remedies for skin problems rely on this placebo response too. Indeed skin problems such as eczema are particularly likely to respond well to treatment that is offered with encouragement and enthusiasm.

There is, of course, nothing at all wrong with a practitioner using the placebo response as long as he does not use it to justify unreasonable claims for fees.

82

Herbalism

Herbalism is one of the weakest forms of alternative medicine. There is, I believe, a cruel irony in the fact that although many patients visit a herbalist because they are frightened of the powerful and sometimes dangerous drugs that doctors prescribe, the herbalist often only uses cruder versions of the same products.

The other problem with herbalists is that they do not seem able to agree on which herbs are most suitable for particular problems. So, for example, in one large book on herbalism there is a list of twenty-one substances recommended for patients with eczema. In another major herbal textbook there are eighteen herbal remedies listed for eczema. Only two of the plants on this second list appear on the first.

Just for the record, I have prepared a list of recommended healing herbs for eczema. You can see what I mean when I say that herbalists find it difficult to identify suitable herbs.

Recommended herbal remedies for eczema:

Oatmeal	Comfrey compress
Olive oil	Comfrey poultice
Marigold tea	English walnut tea
Burdock tea	English walnut compress
Strawberry leaf tea	European snakeroot compress
Lavender oil	Flax poultice
Juniper oil	German camomile compress
Bergamot oil	Great burdock tea
Spinach juice	Great burdock compress
Cucumber	Great burdock salve
Carrot juice	High mallow compress
Beet juice	Hound's tongue compress
Celery	Hound's tongue poultice
Watercress	Marigold compress
Raw potato	Oak compress
Blackcurrant juice	Pansy tea
Lemon juice	Pansy compress

I suspect that the chances of a herbal remedy working depend upon the personality of the herbalist and his ability to invoke a placebo response.

Homoeopathy

First discovered in the early part of the 19th century by a German physician called Samuel Hahnemann, homoeopathy is based on the ancient premise that 'like cures like'.

Minute doses of drugs are given with the intention of triggering off a defensive reaction within the body and stimulating the body's natural resistance to disease. The principle has something in common with vaccination, in which a small amount of an infective organism is introduced into the body in order to stimulate the body's own defence mechanisms to prepare suitable defences.

You can buy homoeopathic remedies over the counter without a prescription – and because the dosage used is very small the risk of side effects is slight. But I do suggest that if you want to try homoeopathy then you visit a qualified practitioner. To get the best out of this form of treatment the practitioner needs to treat not just your skin, but your whole body. Only qualified medical practitioners are properly trained in the practice of homoeopathy and they must take an additional postgraduate course in the subject since it is, as yet, ignored in formal medical training.

When you visit a homoeopathic practitioner he will prescribe a drug which, if given in larger doses, would produce the very symptoms of which you are complaining. To prepare their medicines, homoeopaths, in effect, empty a bottle of medicine into a lake and then use the lake water as the medicine.

There is no real evidence to show just how useful – or useless – homoeopathic practitioners are in the treatment of eczema and other skin disorders.

Naturopaths

Naturopaths follow three basic principles.

First, they believe that all forms of disease are caused by the accumulation of waste products within the body and that these products accumulate because of bad living habits.

Second, they believe that the body is always striving for the ultimate good of the individual and that when symptoms appear they merely indicate that the body is trying to deal with a problem.

Third, they claim that the body contains within itself the power to deal with an illness.

The second and third of these principles are undoubtedly sound. The first is much more controversial and less well founded on fact.

Most naturopaths work by trying to persuade their patients to change their dietary habits. Usually, they will start treatment by recommending a complete fast and will then encourage their patients to leave out certain types of food and to eat large quantities of other foodstuffs.

With skin problems, however, in addition to recommending a balanced, carefully designed diet, naturopaths will usually encourage the use of compresses to draw poisons out of the skin. They believe that when the skin is disordered the whole body needs treating – but that does not mean that they completely ignore the skin itself.

Since we do now know that some forms of eczema are caused by allergies to particular foods there is some reason for believing that naturopaths may be able to help eczema sufferers. However, I am afraid that I still have not managed to find any clinical evidence to show that naturopathy does work with skin problems. It is not difficult to organise proper clinical trials but until naturopaths do this I shall remain reluctant to recommend their skills.

Psychotherapy

Many skin disorders, including eczema, are caused by, or made worse by, stress, anxiety and worry. This means that the symptoms of skin disease can often be relieved by different forms of psychotherapy. The type of psychotherapy most commonly used is hypnotism.

So, for example, someone who finds it difficult to relax and who recognises that tension is a possible contributory factor in the development of their eczema may well visit a hypnotherapist for advice and treatment. The results can be excellent.

I do suggest that anyone contemplating a visit to a

hypnotherapist read the following notes very carefully.

● There are many unqualified hypnotherapists around. Some of them are reliable and honest. Many of them are, I fear, unreliable and potentially dangerous, dabbling with techniques which they do not fully understand. If you want to try hypnotherapy ask your doctor to recommend a local practitioner. He will almost certainly know which ones are sensible and which are not. Do not believe any hypnotherapist who tells you that he is qualified and take no notice of diplomas. There are no formal qualifications for hypnotherapy and some of the so-called 'colleges' of hypnotherapy are little more than shops printing and selling worthless diplomas.

● Some hypnotherapists practise a technique called 'regression' in which they take their patients back through the years, either to childhood or, sometimes, to an alleged earlier life. Regression is potentially dangerous and should only ever be practised by a qualified doctor working in hospital.

● Sensible, well-trained hypnotherapists know that it is dangerous for them to try and treat patients suffering from depression or severe anxiety. If you are feeling anxious or depressed do not visit a hypnotherapist. Visit your doctor instead.

Miscellaneous tips for eczema sufferers

● Keep your finger nails cut short. This will reduce the amount of damage you do if you scratch yourself.

● When drying yourself use a smooth, soft towel rather than a rough one. And pat yourself dry, do not rub hard.

● If you use a bath oil make sure that you put a rubber mat in the bottom of the bath. Bath oils are very slippery.

● Avoid feathers, wool or down in your bedding since these can all cause irritation. Cotton sheets and blankets are best. Or use a duvet with a synthetic filler.

● House dust can often make eczema worse. It is important to try and keep your surroundings as clean – and as free of dust – as possible.

● If you have central heating do not turn it up too high. And beware of gas and electric fires. If the air is too dry that will make skin problems worse.

- Avoid biological washing powders and fabric conditioners when washing clothes.
- Leather shoes are best – they enable the feet to breathe.
- Clothes that contain rough seams or rough patches can exacerbate eczematous areas.
- Do not wash in water that is too hot – this irritates the skin and produces additional itching.

Appendix

I suggest that eczema sufferers and their relatives contact the :
National Eczema Society, Tavistock House North,
Tavistock Square, London WC1H 9SR.

In addition to raising funds for research, the society provides
parents and sufferers with information and help.

The society publishes its own journal and a wide range of
useful leaflets and brochures.

INDEX